The Bite Me Diet Book

Healthy Eating with an Attitude

By Rodney Robbins

Copyright

WARNING

The author is not a doctor or dietitian. If you live with any chronic illness, or suspect you may be dealing with diabetes, high cholesterol, high blood pressure or any other medical condition, please talk to your doctor or nutritionist before making significant changes to your diet or activity level.

Contents

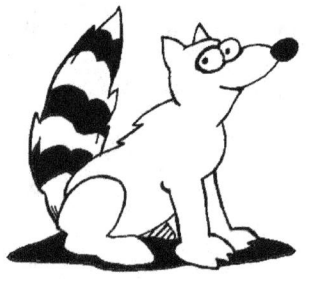

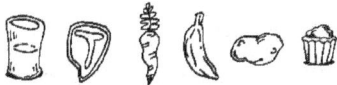

1. The World Can Bite Me

"Do what you feel to be right in your heart—for you'll be criticized anyway. You'll be damned if you do, and damned if you don't," said First Lady Eleanor Roosevelt, American diplomat, politician and activist.

I hate Nice People. If you are nice to them, they sometimes accidentally invite you into their nice little circle of other Nice People where you can talk about nice things like puppies and how clever their children are. But better not bang your knee on the lunch table and say one forking curse words or, heaven forbid, have a strong opinion about anything. And by the way, you had better not be fat, or ugly, or old, or get sick and slow down the pack. Meanwhile, little Miss Nicely over there is banging her minister after bible study on Thursday nights (and twice on Sundays), and Mr. Goody Goody in the sport coat and loafers; he pays the waitresses in his restaurant $2.00 an hour and keeps them chronically short staffed so they can't give good service and earn good tips. All these freaking Nice People can bite me. To hell with all of them!

People who make crap food and write crap diet books are even worse (yes, I do see the irony). Our food today is laced with addictive "flavor enhancers" specifically designed, taste tested and guaranteed to make you eat more of their unhealthy swill. Do they care that we're in the middle of a freaking Health Care Apocalypse of heart attacks, diabetes, strokes, and knee and hip replacements? No. Our colleges are pushing out a fresh crop of non-critical thinkers to replace the old farts like me who are dying off in droves.

Weight loss authors, my Lord, save me from those greedy bastards. "You—yes you—can lose all the weight you want if you'll just stop eating all carbohydrates, cut your protein intake down to one bite a day and eliminate all fat from your diet!" When that doesn't work for you, and it won't, then you are a stupid, brainless, weak-willed cow who deserves to be fat. They can all freaking bite me!

How much fracking damage have these people done in this world? How many innocent people have died or given up on life because they asked for help and were fed a load of rubbish by someone they trusted: an expert, a doctor, a renowned diet researcher? A public whipping is too good for them—drawing and quartering might suffice.

Hey, if any of those plans work, or worked, for you, God bless, but in general, nobody actually cuts their carbs down to the crazy low levels promoted in low carb diet books. People will go lower than when they started, but 20 grams of carbohydrates a day is insane. That's literally one quarter of one piece of toast. Calorie counting? Not possible. Not really. Even if all you ate was carefully measured portions of prepackaged "food products," you could still never, by power of will and careful attention, count your calories carefully enough to guarantee weight loss, gain, or control of any kind. What about low fat diets? They're okay, if you don't mind being constantly hungry, sickly, cold and cranky. (Cranky, you say? Yes, I'm cranky, but it's not because I don't eat enough. I was born cranky.)

Let me bottom-line it for you.

I reviewed over 200 medical studies on weight loss, obesity, appetite, cravings, diet with exercises, diet without exercise and more. If you try a new diet today, the chances are three in five that it will not work for you. If it *does* work for you,

you might lose a little weight—like 5-10% of your total body weight, and then gain half of it back in the first year. So, if you weigh 200 pounds, you might lose 5% or 10 pounds and get down to 190. By the end of the year, you'll gain half of that back and end up around 195. If you are lucky or determined enough, you may lose 10% or 20 pounds and get down to 180. Within a year, you'll probably gain half of that weight back and end up around 190 pounds. That's in a lab setting with clinical support and personal follow-up.

Does that little bit of weight loss make a difference? Well, yeah. In terms of your health, it probably does. Even a 5-10% weight loss can improve your blood sugar, insulin resistance, blood pressure, and your risk of heart attack and stroke. But it is nowhere near the stupendous claims most diet authors brag about. "Results not typical" my assets!

So, what's my point? What's my plan? What Great Diet Revelation do I recommend?

Since, historically, weight loss plans don't work very well, I think we should just eat a healthy diet with a wide variety of real, wholesome foods; let our weight fall where it will, and do all those things we would do if we were skinny.

I say we throw out our scales, or better yet, smash them to bits and make them into pretty murals or Christmas ornaments. For those of us who may need to lose some weight for legitimate health reasons, I say we use a tape measure and medical lab results to track our progress.

I say we go find physical activities we truly enjoy and get some sunshine and fresh air. Screw the greedy gym owners and the billionaire-oil-company tycoons who want us to pay a $1,200 gym membership and drive all over creation to do the simplest exercises. I say we get out there and do anything physically active that we love and truly enjoy doing.

All that personal $hi7 that's bothering us, I say we forget about it. Screw them. Lots and lots of people in this world literally mean us harm. They want us to suffer, pay, and bleed. They like to see it. It's entertaining for them. Send them all to the gallows, I say. Off with their heads! We need to let that $hi7 go. We need to get some rest. Even God took a rest once. Then, if we can, we need to find some people who will at least be kind and honest with us, and maybe help us get back on track with a healthy lifestyle. That's my plan.

"Well," you might ask, "who the heck are you to give diet advice?"

I admit it up front—I'm not a doctor, nutritionist, or dietitian. I've only read a few dozen books on diet and exercise, and reviewed 200 medical studies. I'm not even skinny!

What I do have is a lifetime of experience trying to manipulate my diet to control:

- **Celiac Disease**. Celiac Disease is an "allergy" to common grains, including wheat, barley, rye, and probably oats.
- **Migraine with Aura**. My migraine triggers include getting hungry or over tired, plus red wine, nuts and chocolate.
- **Periodic Paralysis**. PP is a rare form of muscular dystrophy that causes attacks of weakness and outright paralysis. PP triggers include over-eating carbohydrates, under-eating calories, cold, heat, and exercise.

I also have 20 years of experience in quality control, looking out for the customer and making the invisible visible so it can be tracked and improved.

Eating healthy isn't an academic exercise for me. It's something that affects me every single day. This stuff matters to me. What I eat, when I eat, eating enough, finding ways to enjoy my life as a genetic freakazoid—for me, these issues mean the difference between sickness and health, between blinding pain and joyful living, between being able to stand up or having to sit down before I fall down. I do have something to say about healthy eating and enjoying life here in the Savage Garden.

Are you with me?

If eating a generous plenty of normal, wholesome foods while getting out there and enjoying life sounds reasonable to you; if you think my plan might work for you too, please keep reading. If you do not think my plan will work for you, part of me wants to say you can bite me too, but I won't. Reading this far and turning away doesn't do me one bit of harm. Thank you for your time and attention. May you find what you are looking for. I wish only the best for you and yours. I know it's not much, but truly, what blessings I can give, I give to you. Go in peace.

For everyone else who is sticking around, for all of you who want to join me in this great experiment, for those of you who want to try something simple, different, easy to remember and easy to use in the real world, I welcome you. We, as a nation, need to know if a wholesome diet, joyful living and a few supporting measures are enough to revolutionize the American diet.

I invite you to read on to learn The Basic *Bite Me Diet*. At this point, it's still one big experiment, so I look forward to your feedback.

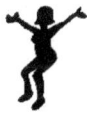

What do you hope to get out of reading this book?

_____

_____

_____

_____

_____

_____

_____

_____

_____

_____

_____

_____

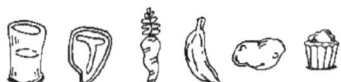

2. The Basic *Bite Me Diet*

"I loathe people who keep dogs. They are cowards who haven't the guts to bite people themselves," said August Strindberg, Swedish playwright, novelist and poet.

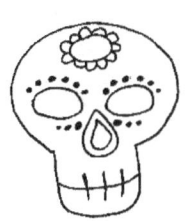 The decorated human skull shown to the left is called a calavera or sugar skull. These artistic creations are a favorite treat for the Mexican celebration of the Dia De Los Muertos, or the Day of the Dead. Catholics celebrate it as All Hallows' Eve, followed by All Souls' Day when they pray for the souls of those who have passed on from this world. Most Americans just call it Halloween. The sugar skull is also the key to remembering the basics of *The Bite Me Diet* experiment. You can use the skull to help you remember how to create a balanced and healthy meal at home or on the road. If you have a little imagination, it's easy. If you don't have much imagination, feel free to write the meal plan on a piece of paper and carry it with you. In fact, in the next chapter, I'm going to suggest you track your meals using a written list, but we'll get to that later.

Imagine a sugar skull image superimposed over your dinner plate. On the forehead or top of most calaveras is some type of decoration: a cross, star, flower, or sometimes a playing card. In that spot, above your plate, place a glass of water. For the sake of

The Bite Me Diet experiment, every meal and snack begins with a glass of water. After the water, if you are still thirsty, you can have diet soda, unsweet tea, or vegetable juice (I think vegetable juice is gross, but some folks don't care what they put in their mouth). The one thing to remember is that every meal and snack starts with a glass of water.

I only have two negative rules in this diet and one of them is no full strength soda, sweet tea, or fruit drinks. Our systems just aren't made to handle that much sugar. I hope you enjoy the irony of using a sugar skull as the symbol for this diet. If you are a working lumberjack or bicycle racer I'll give you a pass on full strength sodas, but everyone else needs to lay off the sugary drinks. Nothing in this diet can overpower drinking that much sugar in one gulp! Sorry. If you think I'm full of it, get in line, but I'm telling you, if you won't give up drinking sugar water, you are pretty much doomed. You might as well just buy some fancy, designer jeans and settle in. Remember, you can be fat and happy, especially if you are well dressed.

Calavera eyes often have flowers, symbols, or jewels in the eye sockets. I want you to imagine a vegetable and a piece of fruit in your calavera's eyes. On your plate, that might be some cucumbers and grapes or green beans and an apple.

The nose of a sugar skull is often just a black hole, but it may be painted to look like a spade or upside down heart. Sometimes, people put little lines around the nose. Think of those lines as pieces of rice. Imagine a starch squeezed into that space. I want you to see some rice, bread, beans, potatoes, or pasta. We're talking about some kind of starch.

Now look at the teeth. Most sugar skulls have big, munchy looking teeth. Sometimes folks will paint pink or red lips around the teeth. In any case, I want you to imagine those teeth biting into a generous, mouth-sized serving of protein. We're talking chicken, fish, beef, turkey, lamb, eggs or (if you can stomach it), some kind of soy burger.

Depending on your size, appetite, and activity level, there may be room in your diet for dessert, but only one dessert per meal. That's the other negative rule in *The Bite Me Diet* plan. One dessert is plenty. So, imagine a little dessert on the chin of the calavera—maybe a cupcake, some ice cream, or a couple of cookies but not all three.

So, water first and always, vegetable and fruit eyes, a little starchy nose, plenty of protein in your mouth and maybe some dessert on your chin. Every meal can be structured this way. The sugar skull visual may be in your brain already, but if you forget, feel around your face or look in the mirror. I wear a calavera necklace as a reminder of the meal plan.

Still not feeling it? Visual memory tricks are cool, but pen and paper work really well too. So, grab a piece of paper and a pen. On the paper, write "Water and protein, vegetable and fruit, starch and (maybe) dessert." Then fold that paper up and put it in your pocket or purse. Even better, make a copy of the list-based food log form found at the end of chapter three. There is also a sugar skull based log form in the appendix. The standard 8-1/2" x 11" format of this book makes it easy for you to copy food log forms and use them as long as you need them.

So, what does a day of *Bite Me Diet* experimentation look like?

Example One

Breakfast: water, coffee, scrambled eggs, broccoli, apple, toast with butter.

Lunch: water, caffeine free Diet Coke, chicken breast, salad with your favorite dressing, apple slices and a roll.

Dinner: water, roast beef with broth (not gravy because, be honest, gravy is just another big, fat starch), green beans, grapes and a crescent roll.

Example Two

Breakfast: water, hot tea, breakfast ham (low sodium is the smart choice), asparagus spears, mandarin oranges, biscuit with butter.

Lunch: water, unsweet tea with your favorite no-calorie sweetener, hamburger of your choice, side salad, apple slices, (you may not need fries, because you had one starch with your hamburger bun), plus a small soft-serve ice cream.

Dinner: water, coffee, fish with garlic and freshly squeezed lemon juice, cauliflower florets with cheese sauce, a fresh banana and rice.

Example Three

Breakfast: water, hot tea with lemon and honey, cold chicken, raw baby carrots with a little salad dressing, pears, and an English muffin.

Lunch: water, diet Sprite mixed with Diet Coke (I know that's weird, but I like it and it's just an example), turkey slices, side salad, Mandarin oranges, bread with mayonnaise.

Dinner: water, hot chocolate (Hey, why not? You had your water and hot chocolate is not forbidden), a nice quiche with peppers, onions and cheeses, lettuce and cabbage salad with your favorite dressing, pears in water with a dash of cinnamon, banana bread.

But what about serving sizes?

Good question. Don't care. Certainly not at first. Most diets want you to start out with crazy tiny servings so you'll get great results the first week. Of course, after the first week, you are likely to have horrible cravings (because you are starving) and quit the diet. I am not recommending that option. In fact, I predict that on the first week of trying *The Bite Me Diet*, you won't gain or lose a single pound.

The primary goal of this diet plan is not to lose weight. The primary goal is to establish a habit of eating a variety of wholesome, healthy, tasty foods then to get out there and enjoy life more. I also don't care about portions just yet because if you drink a glass of water and eat almost any size serving of all those foods groups, you will probably be stuffed. Why measure serving sizes if you don't need to?

Also, if all you have to do to look and feel better is to cut out the sugary drinks, eat some protein three times a day, and grab a few more fruits and veggies, why should you walk around with a measuring cup and a scale? I say start easy, lean into it, crawl before you walk, get started slowly, and enjoy the freaking journey.

But what about breakfast?

Vegetables for breakfast. Say what? If you like eggs, adding veggies is super easy, just throw them in with the eggs, scramble them up and you're done. If you keep a bag of baby carrots in the crisper, grab a few and you're done. If you drink a small glass of—ick—vegetable juice after your water, you're done. If that won't work for you, cheat! Just cheat responsibly by adding a vegetable as a morning snack.

What about snacks?

You may find after eating that much healthy food, you are not hungry for hours. That's kinda the idea. If you eat enough wholesome, healthy foods, you probably won't have room for a bunch of junk food. Even better, you probably won't have food cravings. On the other hand, you may find that when you do get hungry, you turn into a bloodthirsty werewolf willing to devour her own young. So, snacks are good. Don't have one because I said you needed one, but if you find you do need a snack, start your snack with water (remember, all meals and snacks start with a glass of Liquid Rain, a Piece of the River, a little Liquid Life Force), then add a fruit or vegetable. If, after the water and fruit or veggie, you are still hungry, eat whatever you want—within reason. If you find yourself eating a lot of snacks, consider eating more at meal times—especially more protein.

What about desserts?

You can have dessert, but only after you've had your water, protein, vegetable, fruit, and a starch. Here is my only other negative rule: Only one dessert. Not pie, ice cream and cookies. I was in an all-you-can-eat-food-bar restaurant once and saw a mother and daughter go up together and get one of each kind of dessert. They had cake, pie, cookies, and ice cream sundaes covered with candy. The mom was big, but her 13-year-old daughter looked like she was going to have a heart attack right in front of me. Also, you don't get to have a piece of cake now and another piece of cake in a half hour and call that one dessert and a snack. I have frequently been guilty of that little deception! If you have a half a piece of cake with a half a serving of ice cream, well, you're playing fast and loose with the rules, but hey, it's a start.

What about cholesterol? Shouldn't we be limiting fatty foods?

Perhaps cutting fat will improve your cholesterol, but probably not. Strangely enough, if your good cholesterol is too low, it is usually caused from eating too many carbs. The result can be too much bad cholesterol and hardening of the arteries. If your cholesterol is bad, talk it over with your doctor. Get your levels checked regularly as you slowly lower your carbs and eat a variety of sensible foods. See the chapter, Alternate Versions of Hell, for instructions on how to do that. To increase good cholesterol, add more essential fats found in cold-water fish, walnuts, and flaxseed oil.

Three servings a day of protein? Isn't that a lot of protein?

No. Granted, most people don't need a lot of protein for muscle building and repair. The problem is you can't store protein. It is used, turned into blood sugar, or flushed out. If your body needs protein right now and can't find it, it stops looking and just tears down the muscle it was going to rebuild. Our bodies don't have a choice on this. So, what we need to do is eat some protein at least three times a day.

Is more protein better? Maybe. Eating three small servings of protein is good, but eating three or four larger servings may actually signal your body to build more muscle mass. That's good news for keeping us young, strong, and vital. It's also good news for those who need to lose weight—more muscle mass revs up the metabolism.

What about cravings?

There is a whole new field of science focused on food cravings, but so far it seems to come down to three, maybe four, things.

Not Eating Enough

First, you may have a powerful craving to eat because you are—wait for it—hungry! I've seen God-awful diets that tell a 350-pound woman who is eating 4,000 to 5,000 calories a day to cut her food intake down to 1,000 calories or less. She's currently eating more than that at each meal, and some idiot diet guru wants her to cut her food intake by 80%? I can tell you now, my bull-spit detector rings off the chain when I hear that crap! When an extremely low calorie diet fails, and they almost always do, the diet guru or "doctor" is going to say this: "Well, you must be a stress eater." Yea, but that woman's stress is caused by not being able to get her hands around the neck of the idiot that thought it might be a good idea for her to starve herself to death.

If you are getting bad cravings, try eating a little more at each meal. You'll especially want to make sure you get enough protein. Good protein sources are chicken, beef, pork, ham, turkey, fish, or eggs. If you need a number, women should aim for at least 3-5 ounces and men need 4-6 ounces, meat, or fish. That's at least 2-3 eggs for ladies and 3-4 eggs for men. We're talking per meal.

I've also found that when I leave out any of the food groups suggested in this diet, I get cravings. You would think that if I consumed enough calories from my dessert, I wouldn't be hungry in an hour, but it just doesn't seem to work that way. I have never read a good biochemical explanation, but I think the stomach does a little audit after every meal and says, "What? No veggies?" At the same time, eating tons of vegetables but not eating any fruit or not eating a starch also leaves me with cravings.

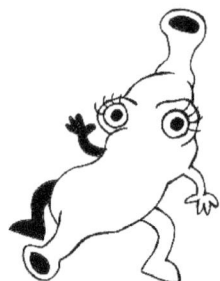 Maybe our bodies are hungry for certain nutrients they can only get by eating a variety of foods, so eating a variety of foods means no nutritional cravings. Maybe eating a variety of foods all at once makes the stomach empty more slowly, so we feel fuller longer and that kills cravings. Maybe eating all those foods together gives the meal a lower glycemic index, so our blood sugar is more stable and that kills the cravings. Maybe it's about the stomach being physically fuller, so the stretch of the stomach walls signals the body to feel satisfied. Or maybe eating "heavier" foods brings more water into the body, so we are less likely to crave water but think we are hungry. I don't know, but eating a gracious plenty of a variety of foods is a better place to start than starving yourself or cutting out entire food groups.

Eating too Many Carbs

You can also get cravings because you are eating too many carbohydrates. I had that real bad for a while. I got tired of watching my diet once and decided carbs-was-carbs and started eating a couple of candy bars every day as my "required" snacks. Well, that was a craving inducing fiasco! I was like a mad man. It was scary as hell to be that out of control. So, if you have lots of cravings and are eating junk food, sweet fruits, too many desserts or lots of starches, cut it out! There is a price to pay for that sugar rush and the resulting insulin spike. The price is paid in wild food cravings.

Stress Eating

Stress is another reason for food cravings. There isn't a food-related fix for this. You're going to need some stress busting techniques—found later in this book—or you'll need to change some major aspect of your life situation, or you'll need some rational emotional therapy. A big stressor for me for a long time was hiding who I really was. Hated it. It is soul crushing and stress inducing all by itself. I blame this on all the Nice People (insert puking sound) and my own freaking cowardice.

Chronic Illness and Drugs

Fourth reason? Chronic illness or drugs used to treat chronic illness. I have terrible sugar cravings as a migraine aura. I have now, finally, duh, come to realize it is not normal to scarf down four Popsicles in two minutes, and that when I get a carb craving like that, I might want to take my migraine rescue medication and a great big painkiller. Cravings can also be an aura or warning sign for seizures.

I've read that food cravings may be possible signs of menopause or perimenopause, yeast infection, PMS, adrenal gland failure and low thyroid issues. If you get a migraine once a month and binge for a few hours, that's annoying, but it's not a huge problem for your diet. If it's every day, or even several times a week, and your diet looks good, consider talking to your doctor. There could be a medical reason for your food cravings.

Some drugs used to treat chronic illness can make people hungry. These drugs including: Prozac, Paxil, Amitriptyline, Depakote, Prednisone, Insulin, and many others. If you think your cravings are drug related, talk to your doctor about switching drugs, using a smaller dose or ramping up to the desired dose more slowly. Many drug related food cravings go away after a couple of months. However, the cravings may flare up again if you change your dosage— even if you change to a lower dose. Weird.

So, pretty easy, right? Not hard to understand, or remember. Water, protein, vegetable, fruit, starch, and maybe dessert. No full strength sodas. No double desserts. Normal foods. Your choice of eating the foods you eat every day anyway. Works okay with fast foods, especially if you bring your own fruit. But there is no way to know if *The Bite Me Diet* is working for you, or not, unless you know for sure that you are actually following it.

Tracking Your Progress

People are notorious for misremembering what they ate. (Sure, yea, that was one Popsicle, right?) You can't honestly say *The Bite Me Diet* worked for you, or didn't work for you, when you don't even know if you were ever following it.

I explained the diet to a friend of mine; she tried it for a couple of weeks and told me it didn't work. "Well, did you cut out the sugary drinks?" "No." "How many days of the week did you manage to eat all your vegetables and fruits." "I don't know." "Did you manage to eat enough protein at breakfast every day?" "Shut up."

We need to find a way to make your actions visible, and it has to be easy. So, pen and paper it is! In the next chapter, I'm going to show you a simple way to track how well you are doing. Then, you'll need to follow-up with someone you trust and go over your performance regularly.

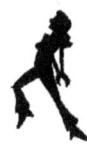

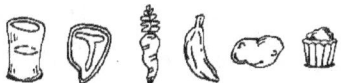

3. Keeping Track without Going Nuts

**"Never discourage anyone who continually makes progress,
no matter how slow," said Plato, the Greek philosopher.**

You don't have to keep a food log to benefit from *The Bite Me Diet Book*. Regularly build your meals using the six food groups may be all you need to do to have more energy for joyful living, and a smaller waist line for better health. If you can do that without keeping a food log, go for it. At the same time, making your efforts visible, easy to track and simple to improve is a powerful tool for getting better results.

You could use an expensive laptop and spreadsheet software. You could track your progress using a special app for your iPhone or Android and hope the battery doesn't go dead. Me, I'm old school. I like suggesting people use affordable, reliable technology that actually works. So, get a piece of paper and a pen. In a pinch, the back of a leftover fast food bag and a crayon from under the seat of your car works too.

Remember, the first goal is not to lose weight, or even inches. The goal is to establish the habit of eating a gracious plenty of wholesome foods and see what happens. The paper and pen are a way to make that process visible and, therefore, manageable and improvable.

I worked in quality control for 20 years. Whenever we had a problem, the first thing we asked was: Did this fail because the process was bad, or because we didn't follow the process? If the process is bad, then we can look for ways to change or improve the process. But, if we didn't follow the process, as written, we knew we needed to try that first.

So, either make copies of the form shown at the end of this chapter, or take your piece of paper and a pen. In the upper left hand corner of the page, write the day of the week, the date and "Breakfast" or a capital "B." It should look like this:

Monday

Month-Day-Year

Breakfast

Next, you're going to add the food groups in a single column. Like this:

Monday	Water
Month-Day-Year	Protein
Breakfast	Vegetable
	Fruit
	Starch
	Dessert

After the first day, you won't need to write out the words. Initials will do. I write my food logs like this:

Monday	W
Month-Day-Year	P
Breakfast	V
	F
	S
	D

Of course, dessert is optional. Eat it only if you are still hungry after eating some of everything else.

Next start filling in what you ate. If you miss anything, write "Miss," then explain why you missed that food. Understand that your misses are very important. Don't skip this step: it is one of your most important tools for making improvements. Write down those misses and the reason why.

Monday	W Glass of water plus coffee
Month-Day-Year	P Scrambled eggs
Breakfast	**V Miss. Ran out of baby carrots**
	F Banana
	S Toast with butter
	D None

Repeat this same process for snacks.

Snack	W Water and diet soda
	V Baby carrots
	D Cranberry muffin

At the end of each day, review your results. If you ate something in each of those food categories, you did great! How did that feel? Did you feel full and satisfied, or dangerously stuffed and ready to explode? If you felt stuffed, back off the portions a bit. If, on the other hand, you were hungry an hour later, consider eating a little more next time.

Remember, those misses are important. Underline them, circle them, or take a yellow highlighter to them. Your misses let you know if you are giving *The Bite Me Diet* an honest shot or not. They also tell you both where you're going wrong and what you can do about it.

"Jeez, I miss my veggies every time!" Better look for ways to eat vegetables.

"Darn it! I always forget my water when I eat fast food!" Ask for a courtesy cup, or drink the water first, and when your spouse gets a refill, ask her to get you some diet soda.

"I remembered to start with water, but I missed having a vegetable or fruit for my snack at work, again!" Consider putting an extra apple in your lunch bag.

The thing is, it is hard to judge how you are doing, or make improvements to what you are doing, when you can't honestly tell what's going on. This very simple food log form will make your diet instantly visible, and therefore easy to review and improve. (Note: An even more *visual* food log is shown at the end of this book. It's called the *4-Day Sugar Skull Visual Log*.)

In quality management, we call this technique a Check Sheet. It is one of the Seven Tools of Quality Control. Making things easy to see makes them easy to manage. This check sheet technique has literally transformed some factories. It can make the difference between on time shipments and customers screaming about late deliveries. It can mean the difference between repeated defects and finding the root cause of the problem and correcting it forever. Please don't skip over using a food log because it sounds too simple. This really is a powerful technique and can mean the difference in how you feel. I want you to know with confidence that this diet worked for you, or it didn't. Keeping a food log can give you that certainty. You can find a basic food log to copy at the end of this chapter.

> You don't have to, and probably shouldn't, use the food log alone. Show it to someone who cares about you. I suggest you meet with your diet sponsor three times a week for the first month. This will help you get on track and stay on track for a while. Let your friend help you brain storm solutions to your misses. When you partner up, you may find that you're not just twice as creative, but three times as powerful. Use that. Take advantage of it. Help each other. Partner up and you will almost always get better results. Use your partner to help you get in the habit of eating a gracious plenty of a variety of wholesome, healthy foods.

Maybe the first day, maybe the second week, but soon, you'll find you really are eating a gracious plenty of fresh, healthy foods. If, after your body has adjusted to this new normal, your blood sugar is still high, your cholesterol is still an issue, or you still need to lose some inches off your waist, then you can make a change. Do one change at a time, and see what happens. When your diet is stable and visible, you can make a minor adjustment here, and a little tweak there, to fine-tune your metabolism.

To make sure you only make little changes, you might consider adding your comparative portion sizes to your food log. You could do this from the beginning. It wouldn't do any harm. If you need the information, it is certainly easy enough to add it into your log. A typical food log entry with comparative portion sizes might look like this:

Tuesday	W *Small* water plus *large* unsweet tea
Month-Day-Year	P *3* thick pork chops
Dinner	V *Big* scoop of broccoli with salsa
	F *Small* apple with cinnamon and sugar
	S *Large* scoop of garlic mashed potatoes
	D *4* peanut butter cookies

That's certainly plenty of food for most people. When you eat plenty of healthy food, a little change, like eating three cookies instead of four cookies, or a medium scoop of garlic mashed potatoes instead of a large scoop, won't spark a huge reaction. Small changes usually don't trigger things like horrible food cravings, weird mood swings, or food obsessions. So, just take it easy.

Keeping a food log needs to be easy. Dragging around a measuring cup and a dietary scale is not easy. Long time dieters can eyeball portion sizes from across a room. They will have no problem writing in portion sizes. If you aren't used to measuring things out, all you need to do is practice a few times. Go ahead and measure out 1 cup of green beans. Dump those green beans on your plate and take a mental picture. Now you know what a large serving of vegetables looks like. The purpose of writing down comparative portion sizes isn't to make your life a living hell. **The purpose is so you don't cut your calories too far or too fast.** Keep that in mind, and you'll do fine.

Without a plan and a food log, you won't even know if you are eating too much or too little. You really can eat too little food to lose fat. Eating too little good, wholesome, healthy food is common. Face it, most people don't eat enough fruits and veggies. Just look at the menu from your favorite restaurant. You might see apple pie or apple tarts, but you probably won't see apples. Apples are a fruit but apple pie is a dessert. We have plenty of people eating dessert, and not enough people eating wholesome, healthy fruits and vegetables. Not eating enough healthy food makes your metabolism slow down. Poor nutrition stalls fat loss in its tracks. It also leads to diet-killing food cravings.

Also very common is not eating enough protein, or not eating protein frequently enough. I talked to a retired widow living on a fixed income. She tried to cut her food bill by cutting back on her protein. Soon, she was trying to figure out why she felt so sick and exhausted all the time. Her symptoms of "old age" magically went away when she added more protein back into her diet. A food log would have quickly shown she was headed for trouble with her diet.

I was on a video shoot once (I have a degree in Music Video Production), and got into a diet discussion with a painfully thin young woman. She said she was tired all the time and wondered if she had Chronic Fatigue Syndrome. When I asked her if she was getting enough protein, she said, "Of course. I eat salad for lunch and dinner every day." I praised her, and asked if her salads had eggs or lunchmeat on them. "No. Of course not. Those are bad for you!" She insisted she got all her protein from the lettuce. Just for the record, an entire head of lettuce has, maybe, 6 grams of protein. So two huge salads a day might be 12 grams. That's not nearly enough for a young woman to feel vital and passionate. No wonder she was worried about Chronic Fatigue Syndrome.

So, you can use your food log to get on track and stay on track. It gives you a way to review your diet, talk about your progress, and review it regularly with someone who cares about you. What do you do when your food log shows you are already eating right, but you still have a problem with your blood sugar, blood fat, or waistline? What changes should you make, and in what order? Find out more in the next chapter.

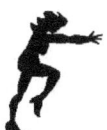

The Bite Me Diet Book Food Log

DAY	GROUP	FOOD AND SIZE	REASON FOR MISS
Day	Water		
Date	Protein		
Breakfast	Vegetable		
	Fruit		
	Starch		
	(Dessert)		
Snack	Water		
	Veg. or Fruit		
	Other		
Lunch	Water		
	Protein		
	Vegetable		
	Fruit		
	Starch		
	(Dessert)		
Snack	Water		
	Veg. or Fruit		
	Other		
Dinner	Water		
	Protein		
	Vegetable		
	Fruit		
	Starch		
	(Dessert)		
Snack	Water		
	Veg. or Fruit		
	Other		

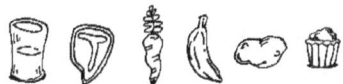

4. Alternate Versions of Hell

"Hell is full of musical amateurs," said playwright George Bernard Shaw.

THE FIRST LEVEL

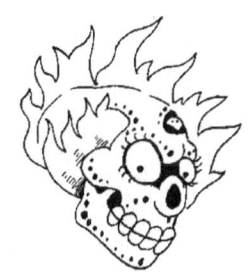

Of course, the title of this chapter is facetious. If this diet feels hellish, you are doing it wrong. Or maybe you just don't like eating plenty of fresh, wholesome, healthy food. That is very much the First Level: making <u>sure,</u> you have enough good food to live a joyful, energetic, boisterous, and passionate life. So, use your food log and make sure you get enough to eat. Every meal should include water and protein, vegetable and fruit, starch and (maybe) dessert.

Who should look for ways to cut back on *The Bite Me Diet*?

If your waist is too big, you might want to cut back. That's bigger than 40 inches for guys and bigger than 35 inches for gals. I don't like to use weight as a measurement because it varies so much day-to-day and because muscle is heavier than fat. You want lots of strong, vital muscle so you can get out there and enjoy life. In a sense, the smaller your clothes and the more you weigh, the better. A tape measure around the waist is the right tool for measuring fat loss.

You might want to cut back if your doctor says you have pre-Diabetes. Normal, fasting blood sugar is under 100. If your morning, fasting blood sugar is 101 to 125, you may have pre-Diabetes. A fasting blood sugar reading over 125 means a long talk with your doctor about your blood sugar. If you have Diabetes, you need to talk about this diet with your doctor or your diabetes educator. Blood sugar is a result of the interaction of what you eat (especially carbohydrates), how active you are, how well your insulin works (or doesn't work), your general health and the drugs you take. I can't address all those issues in this little book, so you need to do it one-on-one with your primary care physician or your diabetes educator.

Same issue with cholesterol. *The Bite Me Diet* is a good choice for folks with normal or borderline cholesterol. If your blood fats are high as a kite, talk to you doctor about this diet and the plan I lay out below for gradually cutting back on certain foods. Remember, I'm not a doctor. I strongly recommend you see a doctor regularly if you have, or suspect you have, any serious health issues. Use the diet, if appropriate, with medical supervision and regular lab work. Opinions are nice. Plans are nice. Lab work is really nice because it gives you the facts about what's working, and what's not working, with your diet and activity level.

THE SECOND LEVEL

If you need to make a change, you can move on to Level Two. Level Two means tracking your serving sizes. I'm not recommending you carry around a measuring cup or scale, but you need to have some idea of how much, or how little, you are eating.

You want to make sure you are getting enough water. So, at least a small glass of water before each meal and snack. This could be as small as a fast food courtesy cup, or one of those little glasses some folks use for orange juice

Like water, protein is essential to life. Since almost everybody knows how big a fast food hamburger patty is, let's use that for reference. Women need that much at every meal, maybe a little less. Men need at least that much protein at every meal. Some people need even more protein. Some people will need up to twice as much protein as the average person.

Who needs more? Anyone who is very active, hardworking, on their feet all day, or struggling with a chronic illness needs more protein. Big people, even big people who look fat rather than fit, need more protein than small people. Why? They literally have more muscles mass and that means a higher protein requirement. Heavy people are also carrying around more weight, which means more stress on their bodies and more effort from their muscles just to get up and walk to the dance floor. Let's not forget that pregnant and nursing woman also have higher than normal protein needs.

You can see how lots of people may not be getting enough protein, or may not be eating it often enough throughout the day. Getting enough protein is not only good for you; it is also a huge boon to controlling cravings. Protein keeps you full and gives your muscles the fuel they need for vibrant living. While it's doing all that, it also keeps you from binge eating on Ruffles and Skittles.

Dietitians and lab techs measure vegetables and fruits with a scale or measuring cup. I suggest, instead, that you log your foods by comparative portion sizes: a large apple or a medium apple; a small spoonful of green beans or a medium spoonful of green beans. Make sure you get at least some fruits and vegetables. The weight and volume of fruits and vegetables reduces cravings and provides micronutrients you need. While having an objective measure in grams or cups is interesting and potentially useful, the real issue for you is this: What is normal for me?

At first, all you need to do is notice how much, or how little, you are eating. Take a moment to write it down. Just include it in your food log and see what happens.

The Serving Size Paradox

The idea isn't to force you to cut back. The first thing you want to do is make sure you are getting enough food and that you don't cut back too drastically or too quickly. At the same time, very few people are active enough to need a giant muffin in the morning (dessert by another name), a huge slice of pie after lunch and four cookies and a big bowl of ice cream after supper. Lots of folks are not active enough to burn off even the cookies, never mind the rest.

The cool thing is that just making yourself write down your serving sizes may be enough to help you slowly back away from the dessert bar. The very act of writing it down can help get you out of the dining room and back out on the dance floor.

I used to work with a lady who was Diabetic. Her symptoms were so out of control that she literally could not stay awake even at work. Her blood sugar was that high! I noticed her eating lunch one day—a huge bowl of pasta with a little butter and tomato sauce. I asked her if it was good, and she went on a five-minute rant: "Do you know what my diabetes educator said? She said that one serving of pasta was half a cup. Half a cup! That's not anything. I would starve to death if that's all I ate." I asked her if she had considered adding any meat or mushrooms to that pasta. "Oh, it won't make any difference, honey. My blood sugar is what it is, and I just can't worry about it anymore."

Talking to her made me both sad and angry. It would be hard for anyone short of a marathon runner to use up all the carbohydrates in that much pasta. No protein to keep her strong. No vegetables to keep her healthy. I had no way of knowing if the problem was her own stubbornness, or poor training in coping with her diabetes. Just sad.

It could be that the magic of Level Two happens because of the Hawthorne Effect (also called the Observer Effect). Folks at the Hawthorne Works (they built telephones and consumer goods back in the 1920s) wanted to know if

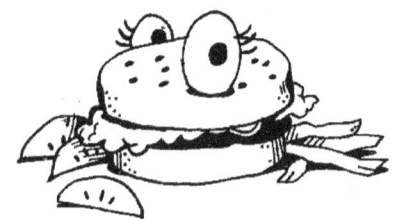

adding brighter working lights would improve productivity. What they found instead was that the workers who were being studied or observed were more productive. It didn't seem to matter what experiment they tried: when management watched the workers, the workers did better. When nobody was looking, production dropped off. Henry Landsberger coined the term *Hawthorne Effect* when he was reviewing the study results in the 1950s.

So, literally, just observing and recording your comparative serving sizes may be enough attention to help you eat a little less.

THE THIRD LEVEL

If you need to, you can go to Level Three: Gradually, but intentionally, cutting back on desserts and starches.

There are four ways to cut back on desserts and starches without triggering junk food cravings:

- Eat more healthy foods
- Eat smaller portions of desserts and starches
- Eat fewer servings of these foods, or
- Substitute a lower calorie dessert of starch

Don't cut out starches and desserts entirely—not unless you absolutely have to! And don't cut out desserts or starches cold turkey! That's a hellish option, and I don't recommend it for anyone.

Eating more healthy foods may mean making sure you get all the protein you need. Remember, ladies need the protein found in a small hamburger patty, a medium size piece of fish, or 2-3 eggs at every meal. Men need a regular hamburger patty, a larger piece of fish or 3-4 eggs. If you are larger, more active, struggling with a chronic illness, or pregnant, you certainly need more. These special groups may need twice as much protein as a normal person.

You might also *choose* to eat more protein because protein helps control cravings. Weigle and associated, writing in the July 2005 edition of *The American Journal of Clinical Nutrition*, found that, "An increase in dietary protein from 15% to 30% of energy at a constant carbohydrate intake produces a sustained decrease in ad libitum caloric intake …." In other words, when people eating plenty of protein could eat more-or-less whatever else they wanted, they ate less food and lost weight. In 14 weeks, the average fat loss was 8 pounds. Those are awesome results.

On the other hand, you might choose to eat more belly filling vegetables and fruits. Vegetables and fruits are heavy and bulky. They fill you up without filling you out. If you eat enough good food, maybe you won't have room for that second slice of Boston Cream Pie.

Eating smaller portions could be as simple as switching from a large piece of apple-crumb cobbler to a medium piece. You might try going from a large scoop of mashed potatoes to a medium scoop. It might be easier to cut back on foods you don't love. Lots of us have habit foods we don't especially enjoy, but feel like we are supposed to eat. I'm like that with French fries. I love me some crispy fries, but most fast food fries are just bland and mushy. I eat them because they come with a meal. It wasn't hard for me to switch from large fries, to medium fries and now small fries or better yet a baked potato.

Eat fewer servings of those desserts and starches. Cake and ice cream. Appetizer bread and baked potato. Grinder roll and cinnamon bun. Two servings of ice cream. Two helpings of rice. These are areas you can probably cut back on without much trouble. Try having just half of the second serving. If that works, try cutting back to just one serving.

Substitutions can work wonders. Find a high calorie food you eat every day, and replace it with something lighter. Instead of a 600-calorie hot fudge sundae, try substituting a 450-calorie dish of ice cream with sprinkles, or 200-calories of applesauce (that's a big serving of applesauce). Or, you could go all the way and switch to 2 cups of popcorn for only 120 calories. At least in theory, replacing the sundae with popcorn should result in a loss of 4 pounds a month, or 45 pounds in a year. Not bad. Especially if that's the only change you need to make.

Women, in particular, may need to substitute low fat proteins for high fat proteins. It's not fair, but men are bigger and more muscular than woman. On average, they can get away with eating more fat and calories than women. So, your husband may be able to eat a big, ol' juicy hamburger and still lose inches. You, on the other hand, may need to choose chicken or fish. See what your food log, tape measure and blood work tells you.

You could, in theory, cut back on fruits and veggies and survive (if you can call it that) on mostly meat. I've tried it and don't recommend it. "What did you have for breakfast?" "Steak." "How about lunch?" "I had steak with steak on it." "And dinner?" "Oh, I switched it up and had some chicken—with diced steak on top and a lovely white-wine sauce." OCD isn't the end of the world, but you don't need to invite it into your life on purpose.

Why don't I recommend cutting back on vegetables and fruits? Because very, very few people eat too many veggies and fruits. It is possible to eat too many sweet fruits, especially if they have a high glycemic index. (That means eating too much of them can rapidly raise your blood sugar.) The glycemic index (GI) of table sugar is 65. Here are some fruits that will throw your blood sugar around as much as, or more than, table sugar:

- Dates = GI 100
- Pumpkins (technically a berry—go figure) = GI 75
- Watermelon = GI 70
- Cantaloupe = GI 65
- Pineapple = GI 65
- Raisins = GI 65
- Apricots in light syrup = GI 65

Pretty much everything else is okay, including:

- Kiwis = GI 60
- Papaya = GI 60
- Dried figs = GI 60
- Peaches = GI 55
- Apples = GI 40
- Oranges = GI 40
- Grapes = GI 45
- Pears = GI 40
- Plums = GI 40
- Strawberries = GI 40
- Dried apricots =GI 30
- Prunes = GI 30
- Cherries = GI 25
- Grapefruit and more = GI 25

Lots of people will sit down and eat a big bowl of ice cream at one sitting, but how many folks have ever eaten a big bowl of fresh grapes or three large apples?

Vegetables. What about vegetables? Shouldn't I cut back on them too, if I want to lose weight? Er, I mean, lose inches?

Basically, the only high glycemic vegetables are parsnips (GI 100) and beets (GI 65). On the other hand, some things that people think of as vegetables, like potatoes and corn are really starches. Potatoes have a GI of 70-110 depending on how you cook them. Corn on the cob has a GI of 60 (not bad) while corn flakes have a GI of 95 (pitiful). If you are cutting back on desserts and starches, you would already be limiting those before getting anywhere close to cutting back on real vegetables.

REVIEW THE THREE LEVELS

- **Level One** is to make sure you get enough wholesome food to live a vibrant, passionate life.
- **Level Two**, if you want, is to write down your servings and serving sizes.
- **Level Three**, if you must, is to consciously and slowly cut back on desserts and starches by eating more healthy foods (especially, plenty of protein), eating smaller portions, eating fewer portions or making smart food substitutions.

If that isn't enough, the heck with it, I say! Eat healthy, get out there, and enjoy your life as it is. Oh, wait. You should be doing that anyway.

WHEN TO MAKE A CHANGE

Your food log measures your compliance to the diet. There are other ways to measure your results with the diet. Compliance and results are two different things. One way to measure your results is body weight. Perhaps the biggest problem is that your weight will vary by 1-5 pounds per day, independent of dieting, water consumption, phases of the moon, or whatever else is going on.

Folks in the 300-pound range may find their weight varies by plus or minus 10 pounds overnight! Weight is an unreliable metric for eating a healthy diet.

Instead, I recommend a tape measure and monthly or quarterly blood work to check your fasting blood sugar level, cholesterol, and blood pressure.

According to a 2004 study written by Okosun and all, and published in the July issue of *Preventive Medicine*, men will be healthier, in general, with a waist size of 40" or under, while ladies will be healthier with a waist size of 35" or under. People with larger waist sizes ran greater risks for high cholesterol, high triglycerides, high blood pressure, and type 2 Diabetes.

Can you be bigger and still be happy and healthy? Sure! Go for it. When anyone tells you different, tell them, "You can bite me!" But if your blood sugar, blood pressure, and cholesterol are high, you might want to rethink that position.

I've met lots of people who want to lose a few inches without it being a big production. Lots of people struggle with health issues that can often be improved, sometimes dramatically improved, by burning off the excess fat that sits around their middle. This kind of fat can mess up your internal organs and play havoc with your blood sugar, blood pressure, and cholesterol.

Now, I don't know how science geeks measure a waist, but I want a consistent measurement that's easy to do when I'm half-awake in the morning, and my hands aren't working very well yet. I measure from the small of my back to my belly button and pull gently. The small of my back doesn't move and neither does my Navel Gazing Place. Exactly how you do it doesn't matter nearly as much as doing it the exact same way every time. When you're tracking results, more than anything else, you want consistency. You don't want to measure your high waist one day, and your sagging belly the next day. Either one will work, just keep it the same every time. If in doubt, measure the thickest part. That's where you will show results fastest.

It is probably a good habit to measure your waist every day. However, give your body a week or two to adjust to any changes. If you make a change in your diet, you won't see results overnight. Even the right change can take a week or two to show up physically as a shrinking waistline. But, if your waist measurement hasn't budged in 2 weeks, review your food log. If you are sure you are eating enough, consider making a change. One change at a time. Take two weeks. See how it works. Make another change, only if necessary. Keep playing and trying new things till you find what works for you.

Don't worry if you start out fat. Don't beat yourself up about the results from the tape measure. "Oh, I'm nowhere close to my ideal body shape!" Being fat means your body is doing exactly what it is supposed to be doing with those extra calories: storing them in case there's a famine. Being fat today means you are descended from a long list of famine survivors from your past.

- 1738 Half the population of Timbuktu in Mali starved to death
- 1770 The Bengal Famine killed 10 million people
- 1845 The Potato Famine killed 1 million Irish men, women and children
- 1876 El Niño settled in and famine killed 5 million in India plus millions in Brazil and China
- 1888 1/3 of the population of Ethiopia was killed by famine and Cholera
- 1921 The Russian Famine killed 5 million people due to starvation and war

If you are alive today, it means your body stores the genetic heritage of living through hard times that killed more than 20,000,000 other human beings. Your body stores excess calories as fat because it is supposed to. Your ancestors survived on next to nothing. Thanks to them, your body knows how to survive on muddy water, tree bark, and fresh bugs. Never apologize for being a survivor.

But what about exercise? Aren't we supposed to exercise?

Anyone who says you *have* to exercise to lose weight can bite me! True—the studies I looked at showed that diet and exercise together work better for weight loss than either one alone. They also showed that diet alone, works better than exercise alone. But the idea that you *must* exercise to lose weight, or to be healthy, is false. On the other hand, being physically active can be a joy, so I'm going to tell you about the best exercise ever! The truth about exercise, weight loss, and passionate living is coming up next.

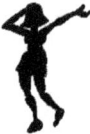

What level do you think you'll start at with *The Bite Me Diet* and why?

_____

_____

_____

_____

_____

_____

_____

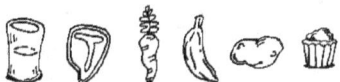

5. Exercise That Doesn't Suck

"To get back to my youth, I would do anything in the world, except take exercise, get up early, or be respectable," said English playwright Oscar Wilde.

If you want to use an exercise like stepping, jogging or walking to burn calories and lose fat faster, forget about it! Unless you are in a biology lab, surrounded by a team of doctors and graduate students, it's not going to help much.

If you've read a fitness magazine or book in the last 20 years, you've probably heard that the fat burning zone is 60-75% of your maximum heart rate. Assuming their guess on your fat burning zone is correct, you still need to do the math working down from the theoretical maximum heart rate of 220, then take your pulse while you continue to exercise without making a mistake, then multiply up to your beats per minute without making a mistake, then make adjustments to your activity level on the fly to get into that mythical fat burning zone. What a freaking nightmare, and, and, it gets worse! If you quit exercising at 15, 20, even 30 minutes, you just wasted your time because this mythical fat burning zone doesn't even kick in until you've been running like a lab rat for more than 30 minutes. You do what you want, but I'm not buying it.

What about weight lifting? Doesn't building muscle mass increase your base metabolism and burn more calories all the time? Sure. Sounds great. I like weight lifting. I have competed in two powerlifting meets. Technically, I'm a state champion (because, hey, no one else showed up in my age and weight class so, officially, I won first place both times). If you like weight lifting, I'm all for it; but coaches can't agree on anything about strength training. The experts are all over the map with this stuff. High reps are best. No, only low reps for strength training. Always go to failure. Going to failure is too dangerous for our NFL 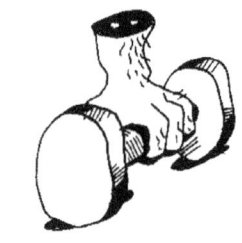 team. Never do singles—you'll snap a tendon! Always do singles—anything else is a waste of time. Everybody knows that powerlifters can only count to five, so we need to take everything strength-training experts say with a grain of salt.

So, what's the answer? Which form of exercise is best for weight loss?

And the answer: You've asked the wrong question.

Exercise, almost any exercise or vigorous activity, will do two things for you. One is to blow off some steam. The other is to keep you limber. That's it, and that's enough, more than enough, reason to be active. Please don't make enjoying life, enjoying the sensation of being in your body, be all about losing weight or gaining muscle.

The two biggest problems with exercise are doing too much, getting sore and quitting; and doing too much, boring yourself into a freaking coma and quitting. I know that for strength training, multiple sets have proven more effective than one set. That's not the problem. The problem is getting so much delayed onset muscle soreness that you never want to look at a barbell again, so you quit. The problem isn't that you are stair stepping at a rate that is out of your target heart range. The problem is doing it for three hours a day, every day, for three weeks straight, till you are so sick to death of stair stepping that you want to puke all over your pretty pink leotard, so you quit.

This stuff does not need to be hard. It is not supposed to be boring. It is supposed to be easy and joyful, so let that be your guide. Ask yourself, at the end of your workout, "How did that feel?" The answer should be, "That was fun. It was almost too easy." Fun? Easy? Yes. Because you don't know, when you are all warmed up, and the blood is pumping, and the pain killing endorphins are flowing, you don't know how you are going to feel tomorrow. Better to just enjoy your workouts while you are doing them.

People die at gyms all the time. Literally. "I'm going to get fit if it kills me!" Well, okay then. Don't listen to the crap from those glossy fitness magazines. The people in those rags are models. All they do is train and eat birdseed. They get paid big bucks to look like that. You and I don't. We've got jobs, families, injuries, and illnesses. Forget that crapola and just enjoy yourself. Live to stretch another day.

So, what's the best exercise ever?

Sex. You get to blow off steam. It keeps you limber. It feels good. It's good for your marriage. It uses your muscles, your physical heart, your emotional heart and, what the heck, it's free! To prevent boredom, I recommend you cycle intervals of long, slow intercourse with bouts of passionate monkey sex. And for you older folks, yes, it's okay to bring some gym equipment into bed with you.

I'm not the only person who says sex is good for you. Kara Mayer Robinson, writing for *WebMD*, did a great piece called, "10 Surprising Health Benefits of Sex." She says that sex improves sleep and reduces stress, both keys to *The Bite Me Diet* experiment. Melaina Juntti, writing in *Men's Journal*, says sex burns fewer calories than jogging, but still counts as exercise. Having done both, I must admit that I enjoyed the sex more.

What's the second best exercise ever?

Whatever you enjoy doing. Whatever you'll do. It doesn't much matter. You don't want something that hurts you, or is likely to hurt you, like jogging for hours at a time, or playing hours and hours of tennis, but short of that, I'm pretty open.

Stress reduction and joint lubrication. Companionship. Fresh air. Sunshine. A sense of satisfaction. Joy. Fun. Play. The question is, would you enjoy doing any of the listed activities on a regular basis?

Activities You Might Enjoy

Basketball
Boating
Boat building
Canoeing
Sailing
Building a kit car
Softball
Tennis (just not all day)
Badminton
Gardening with your kids
Working in your wood shop
Handgun sports
Shotgun sports
Bird watching club
Hiking
Photography
Riding dirt bikes
Walking and watching pretty girls
Walking and flirting with old men
Yard work
Volunteering
Coaching girls softball
Geocaching steampunk artifacts
Plowing your neighbor's field
Chopping wood
Cooking and eating spicy food

Flapping your jaw (while walking)
Calisthenics
Rugby followed by boastful drinking
Yoga followed by green tea drinking
Pilate's
Ballroom dancing
Line dancing
Dirty dancing
Naked dirty dancing
Dancing naked in the moonlight
Bicycle riding
Bicycle racing (in moderation)
Running 5Ks
Mountaineering
Rock Climbing
Orienteering (with map and compass)
Delivering Meals on Wheels
Building a barn
Planting trees or shrubs
Raking leaves
Mowing your grass
Delivering Christmas presents
Putting out Easter eggs
Smelling the salty air at the beach
Taking your kids out on Halloween

Say aloud any other activities you would enjoy doing regularly. Anything that is physically active enough to leave you feeling pleasantly tired is worthwhile. Anything that also has big enough movements to leave you feeling loose, but good, is even better.

SPECIFIC PROGRAMS

Probably because I have Periodic Paralysis (a rare form of muscular dystrophy called a channelopathy), I have a different take on exercise. I'm sort of a time traveler because sometimes my body is young and strong, and other times it is ancient and crippled. So, being able to take the long-term view, I offer the following suggestions on the few forms of exercise I know, use, and have personally enjoyed.

FLEX, CIRCLE AND TWIST

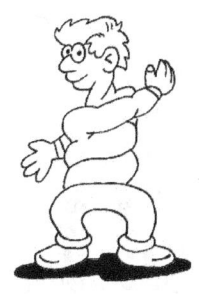

If every other exercise program has failed you, this one might just work. I know that even with my defective, malfunctioning body, I can still usually move each joint through its normal and natural range of motion. I've never been hurt doing these exercises, and they have never caused me to go into a paralysis attack. The motions are gentle and it feels great when I'm done. Here is what you do working bottom to top.

Sit down and pick one foot off the ground. Now flex your ankle forward and back. Circle your foot. Twist it. The ankle joint can do all three movements and doing them gently will keep your ankles lubricated and functioning well. It's also very relaxing. Do both ankles.

Next, pick one leg up and flex your knee. That's all knee joints do is flex, so flex a few times until the joint stops cracking or at least starts to loosen up. Do both knees.

Now stand up, grab hold of something sturdy, and put your weight on one foot. Flex your other leg up and back a few times. Then twist your whole leg in the hip socket. Bend your knee and see if you can do big circles with your whole leg. Don't get crazy. If you don't have much movement in your hips, don't move them much. Only move as much as is completely comfortable and normal for you. Do the other leg.

With both feet on the ground and your knees un-locked, put your hands on your hips and do some hip circles. Go both directions. Then gently lock your knees and repeat. This should really help loosen up your hips and lower back.

Sit back down. Flex your spine forward. Bend backward (not too far). Lean to each side. Then, leaving your butt on the chair, gently twist around to the left and right. No swinging. No tugging. Move gently through your normal range of motion.

Next, twist each arm in the shoulder joint (like you did with the hips) and also rotate our arms in big circles. Flex both elbows. Then flex, circle and twist your hands. Do both sides.

Now, very, very gently flex your neck comfortably forward and back a little (not too far), then side to side. Twist your neck only as far as comfortable and only a few times. Do just enough to keep it limber.

Finally, open your mouth and eyes wide and give them a good stretch, then close them hard and give them a good squeeze. Do that a few times.

That's it. I call that exercise. *Flex, Circle and Twist* is an exercise routine you can do literally every single day, probably for the rest of your life, without fear of injury. Yes, stretching really is exercise.

Too simple for you? Too gentle? Try this experiment: On a scale of one to five, five being the best, predict how well *Flex, Circle and Twist* will make you feel. Commit to your answer and say it aloud. Then go and do the exercises. It only takes 5-10 minutes and you won't even break a sweat. See how you feel. Then rate how you actually feel after finishing the exercises. Be bold. Say your rating aloud and determine for yourself based on real world experience if the *Flex, Circle and Twist* routine is a worthwhile use of your time.

WALKING AND JOGGING

In my humble opinion, the key to making a walking or jogging program work is to go your natural body speed. Just let your arms move freely at your sides. Find your natural stride. Keep it light and flowing. Don't count your pulse. Don't buy a $300 heart rate monitor. Don't make yourself walk more slowly—unless you feel uncomfortable. Don't force yourself to walk faster—unless you find your current pace too easy. Just walk your natural body speed.

On good days when you are stronger, you will naturally go faster. On bad days, when it is cold, or you just have less energy, you will naturally go slower. Over time, your body will adapt to regular walking and find a safe, comfortable pace.

I remember when I was undiagnosed and still very ill. I was barely able to function as a college student taking minimum credits. I walked every day I could because, on so many days, I could barely walk at all. One day, I happened to meet one of my professors who was on her way to class. She was coming from a meeting that had run long. I was, and am, perpetually late. I'll probably be late for my own funeral. We walked to class together, but when we reached our classroom, she was so winded she had to take a little breather before she could do her lecture. I was fine. I had been walking my natural body speed for months and, on that day, it allowed me to out walk a normal, healthy person. (I'll take my small victories where I can, thank you very much.)

WEIGHT LIFTING

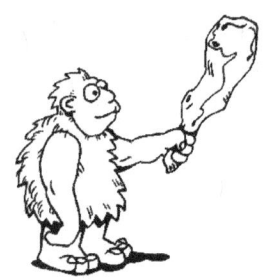

Weight lifting is such a mess. Some trainers still insist that 12 exercises, all done to failure is the Holy Grail. Others insist you need to do 5 sets of 5 repetitions, 4 sets of 8 repetitions, or 3 sets of 10 repetitions. Still others espouse tendon training (very heavy weights, with almost no movement at all). "No, you muscle-bound fool! You need to cycle endurance training, with balance exercises, with strength movements, then move on to explosive power training."

In my not-so-humble opinion, nobody out there really knows how to make muscles grow unless you are a young, strong, healthy, drug assisted male. On top of that, we aren't bodybuilders. We don't want to, or need to, look like cartoon super heroes. So, I propose two alternative approaches that are both fun and probably work about as well as anything else for general fitness, health, blowing off steam and keeping your joints lubricated.

First Approach: Use low to moderate weights and just feel the weight. Let it down easy. Control it. Feel the muscles working. Don't stretch too much at the bottom or you'll be sore. Lift smoothly. Brace your feet. Be stable. Don't squeeze too hard at the top or you'll be sore. The idea is just to put each muscle group through its paces and enjoy the feeling of them working. The result is functional strength with flexibility that will serve you well as you age.

Do 1 or 2 lower body exercises and 2 or 3 upper body exercises. Do 1 or 2 sets of maybe 8-12 repetitions. When 2 sets of 12 reps feels too easy, add more weight and cut back to one set. Your workout could be as simple as 1 set of 10 repetitions of squat, bench press, and rowing. Stop before you do too much. You can always do more next time. The idea is to finish your workout with a *pleasantly worked* feeling. You don't want to ruin the rest of your day, or week.

Second Approach: If you like lifting heavy objects, try working up to a heavy single on one exercise in every workout. This approach isn't for everybody, but if you have good form, you can probably safety lift heavy by starting low and slowly working your way up 1 repetition at a time. You might start at 50% of what you think you can lift. Then work up 10% at a time. So, first arm curl at

50 pounds, then one repetition each at 60, 70, 80 and 90 pounds before trying for a maximum arm curl of 100 pounds.

Your nervous system literally learns to feel okay about lifting a lot of weight. After doing it for a while, your nervous system learns that it's okay to contract those muscles *hard*. Your system learns that nothing bad is going to happen. It feels good. Better yet, working up to 1 heavy single is much less taxing to the entire neuro-muscular system than 5 sets of 8, or 4 sets of 10 using moderately heavy weights. One and done.

On the other hand, if you are not certain you have very good lifting form, and don't have spotters or a power rack with safety bars, best leave the heavy lifting to the guys who take their shoes off to count to twenty.

SPRINTING

Don't like jogging? Hate walking? Try actually running, and I mean flat out! No seriously. You want to talk about stress reduction and burning off the fight-or-flight reflex—that's sprinting! It is not right for everyone. It won't work for you if you are very heavy or out of shape. Certainly, you will benefit from some warm ups, gradually running faster and faster, but here is a simple plan.

Find a spot of grass maybe 25 or 50 yards long. Walk down and walk back. Then jog down and walk back. Then jog down faster and walk back. Repeat as necessary. Then, when you feel ready, run really hard, and walk back and forth a few times. Repeat until tired. Dogs love this, especially in the cold. I call it Puppy Crazies. If you're not having at least as much fun as your dog, you need to make some changes in your life!

Sprinting is your chance to let it all hang out. Loki, over at BodyBuilding.com, calls sprinting, "The purest, most powerful physique shaper in an athlete's arsenal." I just think it's kind of a kick. Personally, I find sprinting is particularly good as a combination of exercise and stress relief.

And speaking of stress relief, some folks do overeat because of stress. Some folks do miss sleep because of stress. Many people struggle to deal with anxiety. Other folks just find life, well, stressful. So, keep reading to learn more about Ball Busting Stress Relief.

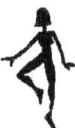

Which type of joyful activity do you want to try first?

_____

_____

_____

_____

How are you going to fit your favorite joyful activities into your schedule?

_____

_____

_____

_____

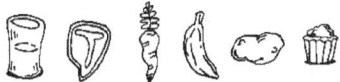

6. Ball Busting Stress Relief

"Under certain conditions, profanity provides a relief denied even by prayer," said novelist and humorist Mark Twain.

This is a three-part chapter. First, I'm going to give you my number one stress busting advice. Second, some stress busting tips, in case one of them is just what you need to hear. Third, some powerful stress reducing meditation techniques I learned from my parents. They ran meditation groups the whole time I was growing up. My mother still does.

BEST ADVICE

So, what's my number one stress busting advice? *Be yourself!*

I have, at times, felt the need to hide my illnesses and stifle my opinions. It has never worked out well for me. It is, frankly, horrible, to be barely able to walk and mentally screaming, "Smile. Keep moving. Don't let them see how slow you are. Stop and fix that trash can so they won't notice you can barely walk.

Ignore the pain. Keep moving." It is also very stressful to be constantly walking around with your hand metaphorically over your mouth mentally whispering, "Shut up. Shut up. You need this job. Don't say it. Keep your flocking mouth shut!"

I can't say that being yourself won't keep you from getting fired anyway. I can't promise that being yourself won't make your poor, poor co-workers or straight-laced family members uncomfortable or unhappy (and we wouldn't want that, the poor darlings are so delicate). But I guarantee you, if you are hiding, you will be miserable, and you will never find your true family. You will never have true friends. You will never be able to relax. You will always be stressed and miserable and working way harder than you need to.

Honestly, I would rather see you fat and happy and enjoying life, than hiding behind ugly clothes with your hair covering your eyes, afraid to move or speak or laugh. If you are quiet, it's okay to be quiet. If you are a plus size lesbian truck driver who is fond of studded leather, I say go for it. To hell with everybody else! Be who you are. If you are a Christian first, last and always, then let that show in the way you love and care for your family and the people around you. Don't talk about it. Don't preach it. Live it. Be it.

Let *who you are* shine so brightly that there is no need to explain or complain. I'm not saying you have to put yourself out there all the time. I'm just saying that if you are hiding, stop hiding, and sin boldly. Be thoughtful. Be careful. Be smart, but be honest.

So, how do you do that? Like everything else in this book, I suggest you start slowly, gently, and lean into it. You don't need to scare the horses to be more authentically yourself. Reveal yourself slowly. Make gradual changes. In fact, you might want to make a lot of these changes in your imagination first, before you try rolling them out in the real world. Trying being your authentic self with strangers next. Go somewhere else, somewhere far away, and try on your authentic face.

Be safe. Take care, if you need to, and be sure before you expose yourself to the people closest to you. If you feel unsafe, if your intuition tells you to stay quiet with this one or that one, by all means listen! Being your true self isn't the same as being your stupid self. Let's be smart about this, but remember, if you are hiding, you can't hide forever.

STRESS REDUCTION TIPS

Exercising for joy is a great stress reducer. Don't do it for your heart. Don't do it for your waistline. Don't do it because an evil little voice in your head says you have to, you should, or you better. Do it because it feels good. Honestly, most people are going to find square dancing with their friends is a lot more fun than doing a 20 rep squat routine till they puke.

Sex, as I mentioned earlier, is a great stress reducer. Even my worst sexual experience was better than my best day working in a factory. I even like sex where I make my partner happy. Try that for a week. Give your partner whatever he or she wants for a week and report back with your results (details, I want details). Highly recommended.

Learning to say no is a very powerful tool for preventing stress before it begins. Here's a tip on that one: Have a reason to say no. "Oh, Jane, I'd love to drop everything and bust my budget so I can cook six pies for your bake sale tomorrow, but my son needs me to help him study for a math test." Then look at your watch and say, "Oh, look at the time! I've got to go."

Tip twenty-percent. Make that your standard tip. Make generosity your standard practice. Just plan on it. You may be surprised how much more you enjoy your meals when you know you are going to give your server a good tip. You aren't busy judging. You aren't worried about if, when, how much. In a sense, even if the service is barely so-so, you 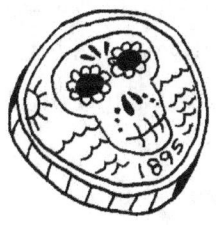 have already decided to give your server the benefit of the doubt and a healthy tip. That tip is well earned.

Forgive, but don't forget. If someone shafted you, left you holding the bag, blamed you, or was just a pain to be around, you can forgive them, but that doesn't mean you have to put your head back in a hornets nest. Forgive the sin. Love the sinner. Just don't give them the keys to your car—again.

Let go of the past. Think, instead, of ways to please your spouse. I've used this one to distract myself from those terrible, circling, mind traps caused by excessive stress and worry. As soon as you notice yourself circling the mental drain, switch gears and think of something nice you can do for your spouse. Can you do the dishes? Does she like cheesecake? Can you buy him a new suit? Did she mention a new book she wants? Can you drive with him to the gun range? Take all that worry energy, and turn it into creative energy to the benefit of your relationship. The bonus here is that your spouse will love it, and that's a powerful stress buster all by itself.

Remember this phrase: "You can fire me, but you can't tell me what to do." This powerful stress-busting phrase can work wonders, or get you fired. It was said by Robert B. Parker's fictional character Jesse Stone in the movie "Thin Ice." This is a very honest way to live. Very manly. Very freeing. Of course, you have to mean it, or you could find yourself drowning in a whole new level of stress.

Give thanks every night. Hands folded, on your knees by your bed; or just laying quietly under the covers staring into the darkness, go ahead and thank God for all his blessings. "Thank you, Lord, for the beautiful sun, and that luscious chicken sandwich I had at lunch. Thank you for my health, and my children who have such strong voices, and my spouse who came home early from work— 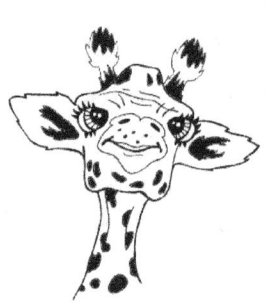 for once!" Hey, I never said you couldn't be a little sarcastic while you are being thankful. I've seen giraffes up close, so I know God has a sense of humor.

Remember, we are the only primates that live in pretty, air conditioned houses with carpeting and Internet TV. We eat food from the other side of the planet. We travel in machines that go faster than any cheetah and have access to life saving medicines that no other animal will be smart enough to invent for

250,000 years, if ever! Even when life sucks, it's still better than sitting in a tree, holding a banana leaf, wishing the cold rain would stop. Be grateful. Say it—even if you only say it quietly in your own mind. Gratitude is a powerful tool for stress reduction.

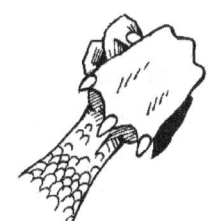 **Confess your sins**. While we are touching, however briefly, on issues of faith, try confessing your sins. If you have wronged someone, be sorry about it for God's sake! I am not suggesting you dwell on your sins. Don't let the Devil torture you with them. If you feel like the Devil is torturing you with your sins, tell him, "You can bite me, you big, fat liar!" But if you have screwed up, be willing to admit it, even if only to yourself. "I shouldn't have said that today. That was unkind." Well, that's okay. Better to try this: "The next time I feel like saying something mean, I'm going to offer to buy the other person a soda and just let them vent."

Have a good cry. Need stress reduction bad? Try crying. People under severe stress are sometimes afraid to cry because they are sure if they get started, they will never stop. But the tears do stop. It might take an hour or two hours, off and on, but nobody in the history of the world has ever been unable to stop crying—eventually.

MEDITATION

Some of the above tips can work great for extreme stress. What about preventing stress from getting out of hand in the first place? Meditation can be a powerful tool to keep you grounded and stable. I reviewed more than a dozen studies on meditators. Results showed that people with a regular meditation practice are more stress resistant and have more stable moods. They also enjoy decreased blood pressure, and have stronger immune systems. People who meditate also think more clearly, possibly because they have improved quality, and duration of sleep.

I believe meditation helps people keep their problems in perspective. When your meditation is going well, your other problems just seem smaller in comparison.

So, let's not make this complicated. Find a seat that allows you to sit comfortably with your back straight and your feet flat on the floor. If that won't work for you due to health reasons, try lying down on your back. Place a pillow under your knees and a folded towel under your neck. Then try one, or all, of the meditations outlined below. Each technique has its benefits and strengths. Keep doing whichever one, or ones, work best for you.

Body Scan

You might want to start with the Body Scan. This meditation is particularly good if you are struggling with a painful chronic illness. To get started, sit with your feet flat on the floor, or lay down in a supported position. Take a few deep breaths and relax. Now, move your attention to your left foot and ankle. See how it feels. Does it hurt? Does it feel warm or cold? If it feels tight, tell your foot to relax, but don't try to force it. Now, move up to your lower leg.

Repeat the same process of checking and relaxing each body part. Go segment by segment, joint by joint. Sometimes moving each joint slightly will help you focus your attention on that spot. Move to above the knee, then your hips, then back down to the right foot and up. Then to the lower back and stomach. Next, focus on the mid and upper back and chest. Then scan down your left arm, then the right arm. Check your neck for tension and, especially, your face.

If you find you don't feel connected to an area, move the nearest joint a little and see if that will help you make a connection. Or tighten the muscles in that area enough so you can feel them, then release.

When I started doing this meditation, I was very ill and unable to work. I thought I hurt everywhere. It turned out, I was only having pain in a few areas at a time. Weird as it sounds, I found knowing that only my right foot, left thigh, and chest felt like they were on fire was very freeing and encouraging. It gave me hope.

Problems? You may find some uncomfortable memories stored in your muscles. When you release your muscle tension, you may also release the memories, and that could make you cry. Most people, I hope, will not have enough bad physical memories for this to be more than a minor bother. If strong memories or feelings come up, embrace them, recognize them and say thank you to those muscles for protecting you from those bad feelings. Tell your muscles good job, and that you are now moving on from those bad times.

Name That Thought

Another weird thing that comes up a lot with people just getting started doing mediation is commonly referred to as the Monkey Mind. Your body and breathing become still, and you finally hear your mind running wild, worrying, chattering, running on and on about nothing and everything. It can be frightening, even overwhelming. It can be shocking to hear the crap your mind thinks about.

"You are a total failure. How could you say those things to that poor cashier? Can't you even tie your own shoes? What is wrong with you? You are fat, and ugly, and your underwear looks hideous!" Ugh! Who needs it? And what on earth can you do about it?

Simple: name that thought. This inner dialog, this inner gremlin, demon, ego, Interject or whatever you want to call it, is a magician who hates to have his tricks exposed. When your Monkey Mind says, "You are a total failure," name that thought: "Berating myself over nothing." When your Monkey Mind says, "How could you say those things to that poor cashier?" mentally name that thought: "Worrying about the past." As for being fat and ugly, name that thought: "Beating myself up for having survivor DNA."

It sounds too simple to work, doesn't it? It shouldn't work, but it does.

People who have multiple personalities often have one personality who is called the Interject. This character has the voice of an overly judgmental parent, a cruel taskmaster, a critic. In theory, the Interject's voice protects the person from getting in trouble. It is, in fact, a powerful survival mechanism left over from our primitive, reptilian brain. (No, I can't prove that, but I'm sure it's true).

At the same time, the Interject's reactions are often out of touch with the current reality, or are completely out of proportion. This trickster tries to protect us, but often ends up making us miserable. It can keep us from making necessary changes—too risky. It can stop us from seeing the truth—too frightening. It can mislead us about other people's intentions—it thinks it can read people's minds and accurately predict the future.

The Interject hates being seen because that spoils the magical effect. Just saying, "I see you. I see what you are doing. You are making me argue a court case. You are bringing up the past. That thought is called dwelling on the worst possible future." So, when these thoughts come up during your meditation, switch gears and Name That Thought.

Problems? Fighting back against the Monkey Mind is easy, but if you have this voice in your head, and you've never heard it before (not consciously, anyway), it can be unsettling. No worries. Almost everyone dwells on bad things from time to time. The more you practice naming those thoughts, the fewer of those thoughts you will have, the less power they will have over you, and the better you will be at letting them go.

When I first started meditating, my Monkey Mind was very powerful. My Interject was constantly arguing court cases with my freedom on the line. I also found my thoughts dwelling on horrible incidents with heartless, zombie doctors who simply would not help me. I relived their abuse, feeling them reject me again and again, as I begged for help and found none. It was horrible.

My first few practice sessions with Name That Thought were 20-minute battles between my Interject and me. I started to see *some* improvement after a week of daily practice, but it took a couple of months for my mind to settle down enough to find a little peace and quiet. Most of you aren't as screwed up as I was, so I suspect you'll do better.

Counting Down

Lots of meditation techniques use counting, especially counting the breaths. I always lost track when I counted up, so I started counting breaths down from ten to zero. I found it easier to pay attention for ten breaths at a time and to have clear starting and ending points.

So, sit or lay down somewhere quit, relax your face, and feel the cool air moving in through your nostrils and up to the bridge of your nose. As you breathe the cool air in, mentally say the number "ten." As you breathe the warm air out, mentally say the word "and." Feel the cool air alternating with the warm air as it passes the bridge of your nose. Count down to zero. Repeat two more times for three sets of ten breaths. If you get lost, start over where you were, or just start over at ten.

Here is the special advanced technique I use when counting the breaths: after counting down successfully from ten to one, three times, I figure I have done my meditation for the day, so I stop counting and fall asleep. Great stuff! What does it mean if you fall asleep when you are supposed to be meditating? It means you are tired. So go with it.

Problems? A lot of folks teach following the breath by feeling your stomach move. Maybe it is my muscle problems, but following abdominal movement always made me uncomfortable. Feeling the breath through either your nose, or your abdomen, is fine. Pick the one that feels most natural and comfortable for you.

Deity Yoga

Weird name, very Tibetan, but deity yoga isn't about deities or yoga. In the West, the word deity means a god, or The God; but in deity yoga, we are talking about visualizing an enlightened being, not a god. Everyone knows that yoga is that exercise you do in a steamy room with a cushy pad, a smoking hot instructor, and a $100 leotard. While yoga can be, and usually is in the West, a physical activity, it can also be a spiritual or mental practice. In this case, it's mental. It's easier to demonstrate than to explain.

So, go to your meditation place and sit or lay down. Close your eyes, and relax your face. Imagine sitting in front of you, or floating above you, a powerful, peaceful, enlightened, calm, amazing being. This being looks a little like you, likes you as a person, and cares about you. You can imagine a woman in white smiling sweetly, or a red demon, heavily armed but there to protect you. You might see the one person in the world who gives a crap if you live or die. Maybe you've never met this protector, but you get the clear impression that your protector honestly wishes the best for you.

You might imagine just the eyes, or just the face, or the whole person, or the person and an entire scene with lotus blossoms and cherry trees, or a cave with rock paintings, or the Panther's Stadium in Charlotte, North Carolina. The

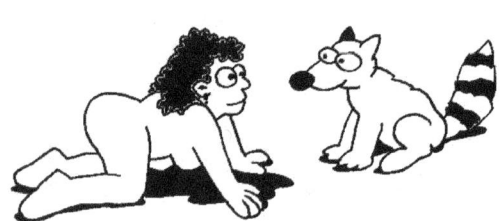

important thing is to see your meditation deity, to see yourself in it/him/her, and to feel this being in you. Hold that feeling for a time, then let it go. All done. Repeat daily as needed.

Problems? Some people find Deity Yoga uncomfortable because they are afraid they might be calling up a real demon or some sort of powerful dark force. Nope. This is just using your own imagination to create a Thought Form. Thought Forms have no reality beyond what you give them. They have no power beyond your power. Anything you see in them, that peace, that protective spirit, that love and compassion, all of that comes only and entirely from you. You see it in their face because it comes from your heart. You may not think you have any strength or compassion left, but if you can imagine it in your Meditation Deity, then you still have it inside you. Take comfort in that.

You can find many forms of meditation to help you fight stress. These include chanting, listening to a gong, bell, drum or chimes. There are group retreats, mindfulness exercises, walking Zen, Kundalini, guided meditations, heart-rhythm-awareness exercises and more. Amazon has tons of books and wonderful audio programs on this subject. I'm going to leave you with one more meditation technique that's easy and powerful. I call it The Wishing Well.

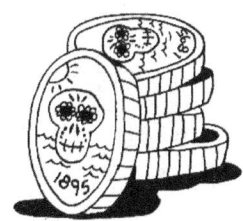

The Wishing Well

This self-guided visualization is my take on the classic Loving Kindness meditation. Go to your meditation place and sit or lay down. Close your eyes, relax your face and take a few deep breaths to settle your mind. Now imagine yourself standing in front of a wishing well. Feel the texture of five thick, heavy gold coins in your hand.

As you grasp the first coin, say your own name, and mentally say, "I wish me well," then toss the coin in the well. Hear the gold coin ping off the stone, echo and bounce and splash into the water far below.

Next, imagine someone you love dearly, someone you cherish such as your spouse or child, and mentally say, "I wish you well." Toss the coin.

Now, imagine someone you love or respect, but in a less personal way. This could be a teacher, preacher or perhaps a friend or co-worker. Say their name then add, "I wish you well." Hear the coin ping off the stones and splash into the water.

Take the forth coin and imagine someone you don't know intimately and don't have strong feelings about. You should feel neutral about this person. Say their name. If you don't know their name, try to picture an individual clearly in your mind's eye—and wish them well. Feel the gold coin in your hand. Release the coin and watch it fall.

Take the final coin and, if you can think of anyone who fits into this category, say the name of someone you despise. This should be someone who has hurt you or wronged you deeply, and mentally say, "I even wish you well." (Personally, I can't help but add "… you dirty, rotten, egg sucking, rat bastard!" Hey, we can't always be chipper.)

You can wish these people well in the generic way described above. You can also be more specific. "Mom, I hope you have a wonderful week in Hawaii." Or, "I hope Bill finds a new job before the baby comes." If blessing your enemies is too uncomfortable, try sending good wishes to everyone in the world. "During this wonderful Christmas season, may all the people of the world find some small measure of peace."

Remember to feel the weight of the coins as you toss them. Hear them spinning in the air. Wait for the echo as each coin bounces down the stone lined well and splashes into the water. Then, when you are finished, let the warm peace of wishing others well soak into your heart. Feel that peace expand out from you to fill the whole world.

Dorky? Yes. Worthless? I don't think so, but you can see the truth for yourself. Use that one to five scale with five being the best. Predict how this meditation will make you feel. Commit to your answer. Then try the Wishing Well meditation for a week, and rate it again. Let me know how it works.

So, *Bite Me Diet* supports include the Food Log, the different Levels, plus Exercise and Stress Reduction. What else is there? Oh, yeah! Getting plenty of sleep and finding people who will support your efforts to eat with love and live with passion. So, put on your favorite nightie or jammies, turn down the lights, and read on.

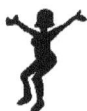

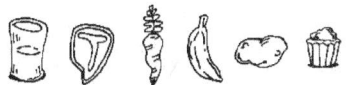

7. Screw It, I'm Going to Bed

**"Man should forget his anger before he lies down to sleep,"
said Thomas De Quincey, translator and essayist.**

This chapter is going to be short because, honestly, you already know this stuff. Sleep good! No sleep bad! Sleep, me happy camper! No sleep, me cranky, bite dog! It's kind of a no brainer, but I would feel bad if I didn't at least try to sell you on the idea of getting enough sleep, so here goes: Get enough sleep! Mostly because it is good for you, but also because numerous studies have found correlations between sleep and weight.

For example, a 2008 Canadian study, written by Chaput and associates and published in *Sleep* found that those who slept too little (5-6 hours) and those who slept too long (9-10 hours) tended to gain weight. Those who slept normally (7-8 hours) had the best chance of maintaining a healthy body weight.

So, make a plan, now, to get seven to eight hours of sleep per night. How are you going to do that? Pick some times and say them out loud.

- "I'm going to sleep from ten to six every night."
- "My plan is to go to bed at ten and get up at five."

- "I'm committed to sleeping from eleven to seven."
- "Not me. I'm never going to bed before five in the morning, and I refuse to get up until noon!"

Pick one. Say something. If your sleep schedule doesn't give you seven to eight hours of sleep, and you feel like you are dragging ass all day, well, you probably need more sleep. Eating plenty of wholesome food won't prevent you from feeling the effects of sleep deprivation.

If your plan won't work on paper, it probably won't work in the real world either, so make a plan that should work, could work, has a possibility of working, and give it a try.

Napping

I love naps. When I was very ill, that's about all I did well was nap. So, nap early, nap often, that's what I say. If you've been out doing yard work for three hours, and you come in to watch the game, and you can't keep your eyes open—don't! Hit the record button, kick your legs out, and catch some Zs. When you wake up, the game will be over and you can fast forward through all the commercials.

The only problem with napping is napping too late in the day. A late afternoon nap can interfere with your normal sleep pattern. So, if you are a napper, do some experiments and see how late is too late. If you are tired late in the day, hold off on the nap and just go to bed early. There is no shame in that.

A Regular Schedule

Having a regular sleep schedule will help your body know what you expect from it. Having a regular bedtime is boring, but it is really good for you, and will give you more energy for living a joyful life. So, if you can, stay on track with a regular sleep schedule even on weekends.

On the other hand, sleeping more can be, within reasonable limits, a good way to deal with stress. Going to bed early or napping late is a much better response to stress than drinking, drugging or mindless sex (mindful sex, on the other hand, is a great way to deal with stress).

A Good Mattress and Good Locks

Buying a good mattress, the right mattress for you, is a smart purchase. You spend 1/3 of your life in bed. You might as well be comfortable. Can't afford a new mattress this year? Buy a nice mattress pad and some deep pocket sheets. A comfy mattress pad may give you most of the benefits of a new bed for 1/10th the cost. You're still going to need a new mattress eventually. Experts say to get a new mattress about every 8 years, but a new pad is a good stopgap.

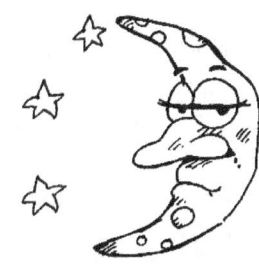

Me, I have a great imagination. I write novels and plays for fun. I'm a natural worrier. I reduce my worries by having great locks on my doors. The frames are reinforced. The doors are bolted and chained. My house is alarmed. I have a dog. You could say I'm overly concerned about personal security, but nobody is coming through my door without me knowing about it. That helps me sleep better.

Earplugs

If you have a good mattress and good locks, you can relax and use earplugs and maybe an eye mask. I started using earplugs when my wife and I lived next to the railroad tracks. Earplugs help boost the quality of sleep by reducing the number of times you are awakened by bumps, cars and screaming cats, or the sound of pizza being digested and other strange noises coming from the other half of the bed. They even work in hospitals. An article by LeGuen and associates in the January 2014 issue of the *British Journal of Anesthesia* found that those using earplugs and an eye mask slept better, even on a busy, post-operative hospital ward.

When I can find them, I like the soft, foam earplugs on a string. The string means they don't get lost as easily. The foam is comfortable and works well. I haven't used an eye mask much, but used to cover my eyes with a hand towel. (Our old alley apartment near the train tracks also had a blinking bar light. Nice place.)

Thermostat

Because of my Periodic Paralysis, cold can leave me paralyzed, and heat can make me weak. Your responses will probably be much milder, but having a comfortable temperature for sleeping can make a big difference in how well you sleep. My solution was to buy a smart thermostat that had digital settings that were easy to understand and use. This inexpensive thermostat keeps my home in a very narrow range of only 3 degrees. I don't wake up freezing cold. I don't sweat to death in a puddle. I love it. Well worth the modest cost, and it was easy to install—I just called an air conditioning company and they installed it.

Lift Weights—Again

A tired puppy is a good puppy. Why? Because they fall asleep fast instead of chewing the furniture. One of the best ways I've found to feel pleasantly tired at bedtime is to lift weights. It's tricky with my health issues and lots of other people will fall into that category, but muscles that feel pleasantly worked leave a person ready to fall asleep. We're talking about the deep, restful Sleep of the Dead.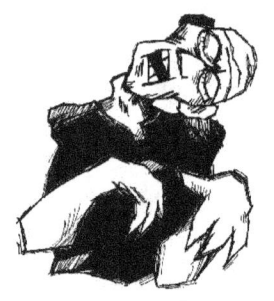

A study done by Rosenbaum and associates and published in the Scandinavian journal *Acta Psychiatrica Scandinavica* found that a 12-week exercise program reduced symptoms of Posttraumatic Stress Disorder, depression and waist size. All that *and* the participants had improved sleep quality. The program included walking and weight training along with standard PTSD treatments. The subjects benefited more when the treatment mix included exercise.

You just want to put some tension on those muscles. You want to feel the muscles working. Make a connection. Respond to what your muscles are telling you. Use enough weight to feel connected, but not so much that you get exhausted or risk injury. There is no need to "train to failure" or "leave it all in the gym" when all you want is to give your body a good excuse to go to sleep.

This chapter is just a brief reminder that sleep is good. But there is still one thing missing in your quest for glorious eating and passionate living: emotional support. You need to find your tribe. You can rake the yard, go shopping, or watch the race by yourself, but it goes a lot faster and is a lot more fun when you do it with someone else.

A group of bears is called a sleuth. A group of crows is called a murder. A group of zebras is called a zeal. A group of apes is called a shrewdness. How can you find your zeal, your shrewdness, your tower (that's a group of giraffes)? Check out the next chapter for tips on finding people who won't bite you in the ass.

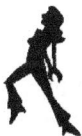

Who are you, and where do you feel like you truly fit in?

_____

_____

_____

_____

_____

_____

Which is more important to you, finding people who share your interests, or finding people who share your values? Why?

_____

_____

_____

_____

_____

_____

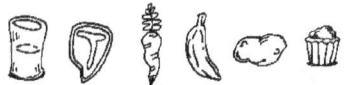

8. Finding People Who Don't Bite

"Loneliness and the feeling of being unwanted is the most terrible poverty," said Mother Teresa.

When I got tired of hiding who I was in the corporate world, I dared to put a Jack Skellington pin on the strap of my backpack. Jack is the hero of one of my 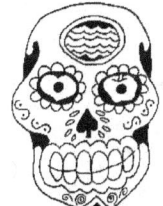 favorite movies: "Nightmare Before Christmas." Nobody at work got it, they didn't even see it, but the pin wasn't on my backpack for three days before someone else did. Out of the blue, the cashier at Subway said, "Nice Jack Skellington pin." "Yes," I said. "It is from one of my favorite movies." "Mine too. I really like Sally!" Sally, of course, is the rag doll who loves jack. Funny where you find your tribe.

Loneliness sucks and therapy is expensive. (I call it "therapay.") When I looked for evidence of the most effective therapy solutions, the results were mixed. Cox and associates, writing in the November 2014 *Cochrane Database of Systemic Reviews*, found much the same thing. They said, "There is very limited evidence upon which to base conclusions about the relative effectiveness of psychological interventions, antidepressant medication, and a combination of these interventions." To be fair, their review was looking at talk therapy versus drugs versus both together in children and adolescents.

I think we can all agree that lonely monkeys are unhappy monkeys. I suspect it is better, and cheaper, to find your tribe, to find real friends, to find other people with similar interests and values than to pay a stranger to listen to you complain. My suggestion is to start by finding your comfort with healthy food and real people.

Where do you find your tribe?

Family can help, sometimes, but talking about your diet and health issues with family can be tricky. Everybody's got opinions, including your cousin Edsel who you only see at weddings and funerals. So, while family could be wonderful for you as you start to eat normally and get out in the world, you are probably going to need more than that. You need to find your tribe.

Can you find supportive friends on social media?

Sure. Sort of. It depends on the meaning of the word "friends." I have friends in a chronic illness news group. I have motorcycle friends on a Gold Wing forum. I have friends I talk to exclusively on Facebook. I do get wonderful support from them. They know what I'm going through because they're going through the same issues. I've received specific health advice from people with the same rare muscle disease I struggle with. I've received specific advice on motorcycle upgrades and repairs, deals and destinations. Facebook is always lots of fun, but I still wish I had more friends in the real world.

One of my favorite social media sites is the one that specializes in taking things out of the virtual world and making them happen in the real world. The site is called Meetup.com. A quick sort of Meetup groups within 25 miles of my house found more than 25 clubs that actually meet in the real world. Here are just a few:

Sample Meetup Groups

- Krav Magna (Israeli martial arts)
- Over 40 Singles
- Survivalist Bush Craft
- Coed Fitness
- Tactical Pistol Training
- Earth Helpers
- Cigar Lovers
- Gardening
- Christian Singles
- Writers Groups
- Real Estate Investors
- Photographers
- Several Motorcycle Meetups, even
- Pre-dawn Kayakers

Joining any of these Meetup.com groups sounds a lot more fun than sitting at home being lonely.

Where else could you meet your tribe?

Strangely enough, some of those anonymous, big-box stores make great places to meet people with similar interests. If you like building things, Lowe's, and other hardware stores have live seminars where you can meet real people that share your interest in home improvement. Same with local craft stores. In my area, Michael's stores have classes on all kinds of hands-on crafts from painting to scrap booking. I think these are great places to meet people because you have something else to do besides talk and, paradoxically, that makes talking easier.

Book clubs, such as those sponsored by Barnes and Nobel bookstores, are a good place to meet readers who love all kinds of genre fiction and all kinds of non-fiction, even diet books. Book clubs are also centered around women's centers, churches, malls, town halls, and local recreation centers.

Where can I meet other people who are interested in a healthy lifestyle?

You might try the YMCA, fitness center, or local gym. There is no guarantee they won't be into some phase of extreme eating or exercise, but at least they're from the same planet as we are. Just be careful if you are a curmudgeon like me: the YMCA can be full of *Nice People*. Most people will like the Y just fine. If your chosen activity is swimming, or a team sport like basketball, you are just about going to have to play at some kind of recreation center or club.

Private gyms come in all sorts of flavors: from hard core "iron gyms" where they wash the floor mats every night with 1.62% testosterone gel, to "chick friendly" gyms where you can't even show your belly for fear of hurting some poor, helpless damsel's feelings. (I wouldn't feel comfortable in either of those environments, but hey, you do what feels right for you.) Try before you buy, and if you aren't made of money, be very careful before you lock yourself into a long-term contract. Some gym owners know more about sales than they do about fitness. If you feel comfortable there, if you feel at home, if you feel safe and welcome, your local gym can be a great place to find your tribe.

Cooking clubs and classes should be great places to find folks who enjoy eating and want to live a joyful life. When it's your turn to cook, you can serve a *Bite Me Diet* meal that's to die for. Nothing in *The Bite Me Diet Book* says your food should be bland, boring, or ugly. I also think cooking is a great way to show love and appreciation for our families.

Gun Clubs?

Shotguns, handguns, shooting ranges, but also any sort of "range," like a driving range, country club, climbing wall, or any other club organized around a specific sport is a good place to meet people. Why? Because you automatically have something to talk about. "Have you seen the new Beretta DT11 shotgun?" "Yes, my buddy has one." Meeting people is just that easy. It's also nice that there are lots of sports where being a little round is an actual advantage—as in soaking up recoil from a shotgun or lifting heavy weights.

But what about values?

Yes. Just so. Long term, finding your tribe may be more about finding people who share your values than it is about finding people with common interests. So, if moral issues are important to you, don't hide them completely for the sake of temporary companionship. Strident hard cases get to eat lunch alone, but if politics is important to you, put a bumper sticker on your car. Mine says, "Independent thinker, voter, believer." (I also like the one that says, "I'm patrioticker than you!") If you are religious, a tasteful piece of jewelry is cheap advertising. If you are a fan of adoption, put a button about it on your purse. If you belong to a fraternity or sorority, get a Greek ring or earrings. Mensa membership? They have a new zombie t-shirt. The back says Mensa and the front reads, "We want brains!" Now that's cool.

Whether you hate fracking, or hate being dependent on Middle East oil, adults should be able to have respectful conversations about important issues without resorting to name calling or shunning. If you get shunned for who you are, for having the slightest hint of an opinion, or for respectfully disagreeing, you need to move on. Seriously. That club or job is not going to work out for you. I've been there and it fracking sucks! Stop kidding yourself. Stop paying dues. Find something else to do on Thursday nights. Update your resume and start sending it out. If you can't be honest about who you are, you will be miserable. If you make your true self invisible so you can fit in, your tribe will never see you.

But what about finding someone to be my diet sponsor?

Excellent question! Jungsun and associates, writing in the February 2007 issue of the *Yonsie Medical Journal* found that people who meet regularly to review their diet progress, those who meet for a longer period, and those who were more highly motivated lost the most weight. I believe that people, who meet with a diet sponsor, double their problem-solving IQ. Hey, two average folks with 100 IQ points each, working together have a way-beyond-genius IQ of 200.

Of course, you also want someone who understands the program, but you can explain what you need from your "sponsor" in about 2 minutes. Use the cheat-sheet on the next page:

Bite Me Diet Cheat-Sheet

The Bite Me Diet is based on eating a generous plenty of water (first) and protein, vegetables and fruits, starches and (maybe) dessert.

There are two negative rules:

- No full strength soda, fruit juice or sweet tea, and
- Only one dessert per meal

Biters track their progress in a food log. Misses are recorded and analyzed.

There are three Levels:

- Level One means making sure you get enough real, wholesome healthy food, especially, getting enough protein
- Level Two, if necessary for health reasons, means writing down comparative serving sizes (small-medium-large)
- Level Three involves slowly cutting back on desserts, starches and overly sweet fruits

Dietary supports include joyful exercise, stress relief, getting plenty of sleep and finding your tribe.

Biters meet with (or call) their sponsor regularly:

- Three times per week for the first month.
- Twice a week for the second month
- At least once per week for the third month

If *The Bite Me Diet* hasn't started to work in 3 months, try working with a professional dietitian or nutritionist to help you see what you are missing.

Your sponsor could be a family member, friend, coworker, or co-dieter. Find someone who is willing to support you on THIS diet. Don't work with someone who will nag you to switch to a nutty diet based on grapefruits, cleansing or not eating entire food groups like carbs, protein, or fat.

There is nothing wrong with starting a *Bite Me Diet Book Club*. You could meet weekly and support each other. Often churches, recreation centers, even hospitals and some companies have meeting rooms available for local users. Use the *Bite Me Diet Book Club* to celebrate your results and share your tips. You can ask each other for help with specific problems like, "Who knows a quick dessert that isn't too filling?" or "Is anyone else having trouble fitting protein into their breakfast schedule?"

Support Groups

Of course, there are already support groups dedicated to weight loss and healthy eating. The Grandmamma of weight loss clubs is probably Taking Off Pounds Sensibly—commonly known as TOPS. They don't endorse any particular weight loss plan, but promote good nutrition, exercise, motivation, and wellness. TOPS has more than 125,000 members and multiple groups in every state in the USA and every province in Canada. The yearly fee is about what you might expect to pay for a magazine subscription. Local chapters may also charge a token monthly fee.

Other groups include Overeaters Anonymous, Food Addicts Anonymous, not to be confused with Food Addicts in Recovery Anonymous. These are all 12-step type programs.

Any one of these groups might be the right group for you, depending on who's in charge, who all is in the group, and where you are located.

Doctors

In my non-medical opinion, if you are making significant changes to your diet and exercise, you should get blood work done at least every three months (quarterly) until you are comfortable with the diet. If you have any health issues, or live with any chronic illness, you should probably follow up more frequently. Again, not a doctor or nutritionist, but in my humble opinion, Diabetics should check their blood sugar at least daily on a planned schedule. Talk to your doctor or diabetes educator about a daily self-testing schedule that alternates your blood glucose checks between morning fasting, before meals, after meals and before bed. That way, in a month, you and your team will have plenty of information to work with toward improving your blood sugar control.

I suggest you to ask your doctor to check your cholesterol regularly. Normal for total cholesterol is below 200 mg/dl. You certainly want your blood pressure below 160/100. The most important body measurement is your waist size. Ideally, men should be 40" or under at the largest point. Women should be 35" or under. Don't be afraid to measure the thickest part of your waist. That's where you will see results the fastest.

That's most of what I know that can help you. I'm sure I've forgotten something. Check out the next section for answers to frequently asked questions.

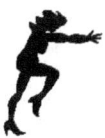

List three people who will support your efforts toward eating a healthy diet and enjoying the hell out of life.

_____

_____

_____

List three groups you could visit to look for your tribe.

_____

_____

_____

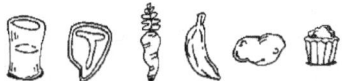

9. FAQ Frequently Asked Questions

"The art and science of asking questions is the source of all knowledge," said Adolf Berle, author, lawyer, and member of Franklin Roosevelt's Brain Trust.

As I've explained this diet to my friends, a few questions keep coming up. If you have a question, the answer may be here for you.

Most diets recommend high priced snack bars or shakes. What do you recommend?

I recommend you supplement your diet with fish on Fridays. Several studies (including a literature review by Mozaffarian and Rimm for *JAMA* in October 2006) found those who eat fish once or twice per week have much lower rates of heart attack.

On the other hand, if you live with Celiac Disease or some other digestive disorder, or just feel like you want a little insurance, I recommend an el cheapo general-purpose multi-vitamin and separate multi-mineral. You can buy these at GNC, CVS, Walmart, or your local drug store. On this diet, you should be getting plenty of micronutrients. I'd rather see you spend your money on real food, like a nice dinner out, instead of expensive supplements.

What about snack bars? Are they just desserts?

Fruits and vegetables are healthy snacks. Fancy high protein fitness bars? Not so much. I call them desserts. When you read the nutrition label on a high protein "snack bar," it reads an awful lot like a candy bar. Real candy bars, pastries, cinnamon rolls and other sweets can vary widely in their nutritional composition and calorie count. On the other hand, they are all mostly sugar and fat. Sweets, in moderation, and after eating plenty of wholesome foods, are not necessarily evil. If you need the calories, they've got to come from somewhere. On the other hand, if you are losing blood sugar control, or need to reduce your waist size, snacks and desserts are a good place to start cutting back.

I've eaten all my healthy foods, but I'm still hungry before I go to bed?

This happens to me too. I think it's boredom—TV does that to me. (Where have all the good science fiction shows gone?) If you are still hungry after dinner, try working the plan and have a glass of water and a vegetable or fruit. If you are still hungry after that, consider popcorn instead of a bowl of ice cream or a honkin' huge piece of cake. Popcorn is filling and low calorie. It is possible that if all you did on this diet was substitute 2 cups of popcorn for 1 high calorie dessert every night, you would lose so many inches the Centers for Disease Control would give you a metal.

I'm a very visual person. Do you have any video to explain this more clearly?

I'm thinking of creating some YouTube.com videos. Drop me a line with suggestions of what you would like to see.

Why haven't you talked about weight loss drugs?

I am not a doctor. I can't prescribe drugs. If you have questions about weight loss drugs, talk to your doctor. I can tell you that some drugs reduce appetite (Lorcaserin/Belviq), increase metabolism (Caffeine) or block the release or absorption of fat or glucose (Orlistat/Xenical/Alli and Metformin/Glucophage). All diet drugs are costly and some have troubling side effects. I think of drugs as power tools: sometimes an electric saber saw really is the right tool for the job. Just be careful with it.

What about herbal appetite suppressants?

There are a million of 'em out there. Some of them work. Many of them that claim to be pure-this or pure-that actually have secret additives like sibutramine. Sibutramine is an amphetamine-like drug that many countries banned because it can cause heart attacks or strokes. If it's in there, it won't be on the label. I am very leery of weight loss herbal remedies and don't recommend them.

The only all natural appetite suppressant I feel comfortable recommending is cold milled flaxseed. Cold milled flaxseed is a fiber supplement that naturally includes essential Omega-3 fatty acids (a healthy fat that's good for your brain). In May 2013, Hutchins and associates published an article about milled flaxseed in *Nutrition Journal*. They found 13 grams per day helped obese men and women with pre-Diabetes get better control of their glucose levels. Ibrugger and associates, writing in the April 2012 issue of *Appetite*, found a low dose of flaxseed fiber "significantly suppresses appetite and energy intake."

Mix cold milled flaxseed with oatmeal, applesauce, cottage cheese, or soup. I like it in my morning protein shake and in yogurt before dinner. You should be able to find it in health food stores, or for less money in the alternative flours section of your grocery stores. For best results, keep the container tightly sealed and refrigerated.

What about bariatric surgery?

The studies I reviewed said that bariatric surgery was effective for those with a lot of weight to lose. For those people, it may be more effective (but much more costly) than diet and exercise. However, it would not be my first choice. I'd much rather eat a wide variety of lush, delightful foods and go dancing, bowling and hiking more often. On the other hand, if it was a choice of two knee replacements and thrice daily insulin shots for the rest of my life, or getting a gastric sleeve—I'd go with the gastric sleeve.

What about dairy? You don't even mention dairy in this plan.

Some diet experts recommend dairy products as a good source of calcium. I'm not certain. No other adult mammal on the entire planet drinks milk. If you are an adult who likes milk, and your stomach can still handle it, I recommend you have a glass of water first before drinking your milk. If by "dairy," you mean a milk shake or ice cream, count that as dessert.

Why does your *Bite Me Diet* book cost so much?

This book costs less than a nice steak dinner, while offering a lifetime plan for healthy eating and joyful living. I don't think that's expensive. It's short and to the point, so you don't have to wade through a load of horse hockey to get to the good stuff. I'm biased, but that sounds like a good value to me.

You said you have migraines. What are some migraine food triggers?

There are whole bunches of foods that *can* or might cause migraines. Even if you have migraines, most of those trigger foods won't apply to you. The important thing is to know *your* migraine trigger foods. Mine are red wine, chocolate, and peanuts. The confusing part is that only the red wine will *always* trigger a headache. The other two are only triggers when I have other migraine stressors stacked up together. My other stressors include: getting over tired or over sleeping, weather changes, too much stress or excitement, eating too many carbs or making any big changes in my carbohydrate consumption.

Will you ever have *Bite Me Diet* retreats?

Maybe one day. As a longtime resident of North Carolina, I know I can easily drive to the beach or the mountains. If you would like to know more, stay in touch through the website or subscribe to my free email newsletter.

- Website: *TheBiteMeDiet*.com
- Ezine: TinyLetter.com/RodneyRobbins

What about Celiac Disease? Is it hard to manage Celiac Disease on *The Bite Me Diet*?

Yes and no. It's not as if you have a choice about it. If you are Celiac, most common grains are literally poison to you. On the other hand, there are all kinds of food in the world, and only four grains we can't eat. Now, more than ever, folks with Celiac Disease can find a wide range of gluten free breads, pastas, crackers, snacks, and desserts. Nobody said you have to eat grains. You can easily switch from grains to other starches like beans, potatoes or 100% corn meal.

One word of caution: If you even think you might have Celiac Disease, or a wheat allergy, do not stop eating wheat! Instead, talk to your doctor and get the blood test first, then think about stopping the wheat. Why? If you stop eating wheat before the blood test, you will stop producing antigens to wheat and your blood test may come back negative when you are, in fact, allergic. So, test first, stop eating wheat second.

Most people do not need to go gluten free. If you are not Celiac, going gluten free is not going to do anything for you except drain money from your wallet.

What about eating fast food?

I have no problem with fast food or eating out. Busy people gotta eat! Of course, you are going to start with water, and avoid the full-sugar sodas. To healthify your fast food meals even further, choose either the hamburger bun, or the fries. Bun and fries makes two starches, and you probably don't need both. The tricky part is the fruit. Some fast food joints sell expensive little bags of apple slices. What do you normally do if you have a miss at a meal? You make it up later with a healthy snack. So, have lunch without guilt, then later, enjoy your fruit or vegetable as a snack.

What about serving sizes? Calories count, ya idjit!

People are going to eat what their appetite requires. Big guys with big appetites are going to eat larger portions, and in fact need larger portions, compared to skinny girls with tiny frames. We all need to eat a wide range of healthy, wholesome foods. I believe that people who eat a gracious plenty of healthy foods will find they have fewer cravings than they used to. They will automatically learn to eat appropriate portions.

I also don't believe in making rules that can't be enforced. I've only met one person in my entire life who brought a measuring cup to dinner, and she was desperately ill (kidney failure) and on a special diet. There is no way I'm going to say that you, or anyone else on a normal diet, need to weigh and measure every bite of food that goes in your mouth. Eyeballing portions as "a little," "some" and "a lot" is fine for most folks.

I should add a note here that men can probably get away with eating more fatty proteins like beef, while women may need to eat more low fat proteins like chicken or fish. Sorry ladies, men are bigger, have more muscle mass, and may need the extra calories to keep from getting hungry and binging. You ladies, on the other hand, may end up with less animal fat clogging up your arteries.

Gas! How come I'm suddenly tooting like a steam engine?

Any time you change your diet, especially by adding fibrous vegetables and fruits, you can get bloating and gas. It takes the body time to manufacture enough enzymes to digest these tougher foods. Go slow. Add new foods a little at a time. On the other hand, certain foods give a lot of people gas. Some of the most common gas-producing foods are onions, broccoli, cabbage, prunes, and apples. Starches don't bother most people, but some folks will not do well with beans or (rarely) bread, pasta or anything made with wheat or even corn. Rice, on the other hand, is usually safe.

Do you offer any *Bite Me Diet* swag?

This diet is just begging for a t-shirt, isn't it? "You don't like my diet? You can bite me!" Or maybe one that reads: "Biters cook with love, and eat with passion!" One day soon, I hope to offer shirt and cool calavera sugar skull necklaces. Check back frequently at *TheBiteMeDiet*.com.

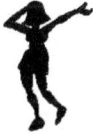

Who do you know that could benefit from reading this book?

_____

_____

_____

_____

_____

What questions do you have about healthy eating and joyful living? (Contact the author at TheBiteMeDiet.com.)

_____

_____

_____

_____

_____

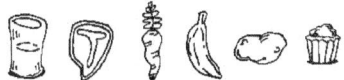

10. Final Advice

Be kind to yourself. Take it easy. Lean into this program. *The Bite Me Diet* is the only diet book I know of that both encourages you to eat healthy and to make changes gradually.

This is your life. I want you to have all the fuel and nutrition you need to live it with passion and joy. I want you to have the facts about what is working for you and what isn't working. I want you to be strong, limber, and well rested for the long term. I want you to live joyfully not fretfully, and to act from a position of strength not stress. I hope you will find your tribe and a place where you can fit in and feel safe, valued, and involved.

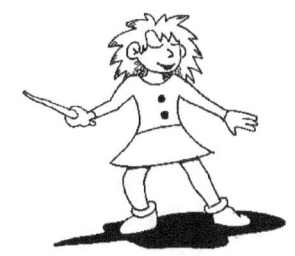

If anyone tries to stop you, or reign in the new, healthier, happier, and more joyful you, I suggest you smile, and in your sweetest voice say, "Well, bless your heart." For those of you unlucky enough to live somewhere else besides the Carolinas, that phrase is a nice way of telling someone, "You can bite me!"

Sing—badly, play hard, and when you are tired—sleep late. Listen to good music with your friends. Eat well. Cook with love. Eat with passion. Be kind to yourself and those you care about. Dance like a wild thing—especially when the moon is full. Then, then my friend, then you have a life worth living!

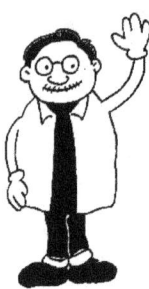

***

Thank you for reading all the way through to the end.

If you enjoyed *The Bite Me Diet Book: Healthy Eating with an Attitude*, if you found it useful, please write a review at Amazon.com. Your review could make a huge difference to someone who is struggling to find a sensible eating plan.

You can also stay in touch through Facebook.com. Just search for *The Bite Me Diet Group*.

Write Your Plan to Implement *The Bite Me Diet*

_____

_____

_____

_____

_____

_____

_____

_____

_____

_____

_____

_____

_____

_____

_____

Quarterly Blood Work on *The Bite Me Diet*

Patient Name:	
Doctor Name:	
Day/Date Fasting Blood Glucose Total Cholesterol Blood Pressure Weight Waist Plan	Day/Date Fasting Blood Glucose Total Cholesterol Blood Pressure Weight Waist Plan
Day/Date Fasting Blood Glucose Total Cholesterol Blood Pressure Weight Waist Plan	Day/Date Fasting Blood Glucose Total Cholesterol Blood Pressure Weight Waist Plan
Notes	

The Bite Me Diet Grocery Shopping List

Drinks	Proteins

Vegetables	Fruits

Starches	Desserts/Dairy

Paper/Plastic Products	Household Products

Condiments/Spices	Other/Misc.

4 -Day Sugar Skull Visual Log

Color over the letters after you complete each meal.	Misses will be clearly visible.	Use snacks to make up for any misses.
Day/Date		